Treasures

by the students of
Rutherford County

Wax Family Printing, LLC
Murfreesboro, TN

Published by Wax Family Printing, LLC
www.waxfamilyprinting.com

ISBN 0-9815604-0-7 Paperback

Title: Treasures, multiple authors.
Subject: Literary Collections, Poetry.

Project Sponsor:
Rutherford County Tennessee Board of Education
Harry Gill, Jr., Director of Schools

Project Coordinators:
Shelia Bratton, Middle Level Coordinator
Elizabeth Church, Language Arts Instructional Specialist
Jackie Drake, Administrative Assistant

For Wax Family Printing:
Publisher: Kevin Wax
Editor: Kevin Wax
Inside Layout: Angel Pardue

Cover Art: Laney Humphrey, Siegel High School, Grade 11
Back Cover Art: Maia Lewis, Holloway High School, Grade 10
Inside Cover Art: Markie Smith, Oakland High School, Grade 12

To publish a book for your school or non-profit organization that complements
your academic goals or values, vision and mission, please contact:

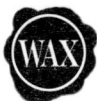

Wax Family Printing, LLC
215 MTCS Drive
Murfreesboro, TN 37129

phone: 615-893-4290
fax: 615-893-4295
www.waxfamilyprinting.com

Table of Contents

Chapter Two
Treasures of Friendship

Chapter Three
Performing Treasures

Chapter Six
Treasured Memories

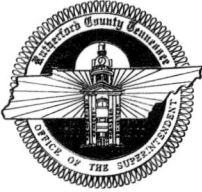

February 15, 2008

Dear Reader,

Treasures, the ninth book in a series of student books published by
Rutherford County, highlights the outstanding writings and artwork by
our K-12 students. It is a collection of stories, poems, letters, and illus-
trations, which reveal treasures both seen and unseen in the lives and
families of our students.

The artwork and writings are true treasures in their own right, sharing a
special memory, time, or thought that touches us deeply. For Zachary
Shugan his treasure of family is priceless; Micah Haskins treasures the
complete joy experienced before, during, and after her dance recital; and
the special Christmas tradition of Krystals and taco soup is treasured by
Jack Jones.

As you read, I hope you will be reminded of the treasures of life found
within your own heart.

Best regards,

Harry Gill, Jr.
Director of Schools

Moving Beyond Excellence

x

Chapter One

Life's Treasures

Soldiers

Luke Hicks
Eagleville School, Grade 3

Soldiers serve our county.
They are great.
They get up before dawn,
And stay up so late.

The war is not over.
They fight nights and days.
They still serve our nation.
They are our greatest treasures always.

My Poem about the Things I Have Learned

Kiera Phillips
LaVergne Lake Elementary, Grade 4

There's more to me than meets the eye, I'm beginning to understand.
It's what I think and how I feel that make me what I am.
Why do I say the things I say? What is important, and how do I tell?
I'm learning more each day.
I learn from friends and family, from work, from play, from school.
I've also learned to take some time to sit and think things through.
The more I learn, the more I grow,
And then the more I see, just how much more I want to know,
THE ME I'M LEARNING TO BE!

Treasures

Daniel Kim
Siegel Middle School, Grade 7

Books are a treasure
That will dwell in your heart
For eternity

When you open a book
Something magical happens
Which many have yet to see

Many other things
Could give you pleasure
For the present hour

Yet books will give you a
Wealth of knowledge
That will stay with you forever

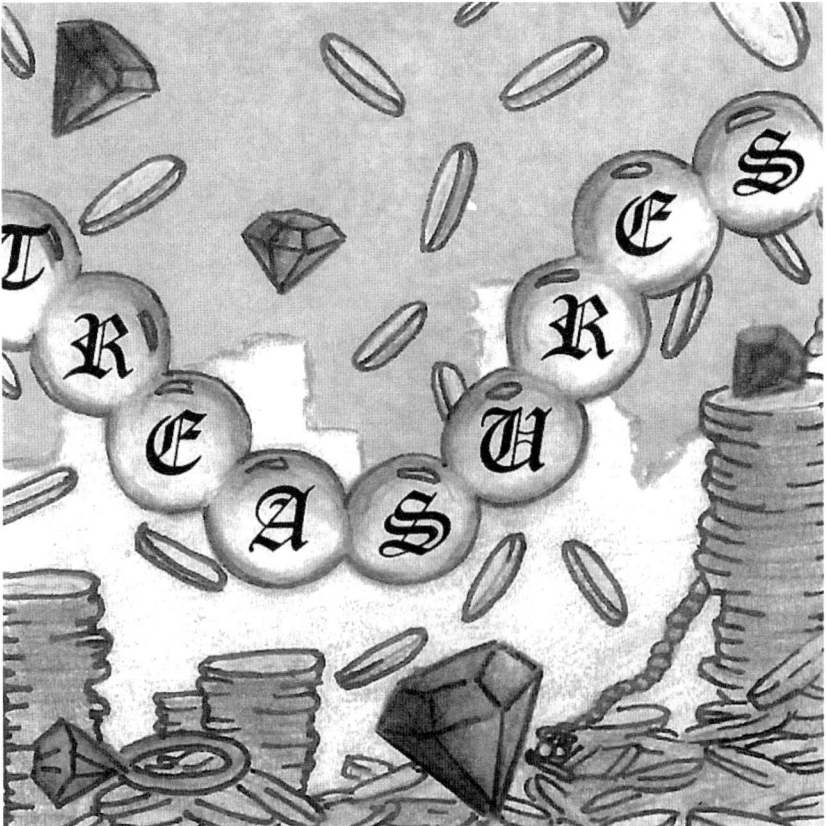

Morgan Taylor, Siegel High School, Grade 12

Math

Courtney Wright
Christiana Middle School, Grade 7

Mode, median, mean
There is no end
Numbers are lines
They never end

I can't be abashed
I'm much too intelligent
Ratios and ranges
I can do blindfolded

Throw me an equation
I can tell you the answer
Quick as lightning

I'm meticulous
With my math
It never makes me vile
You can't dissuade me from doing it

I always feel exuberant
With my math at hand
I'm never reprimanded
For bad grades

Math keeps going and going
Building and adding on
'Yil the building is complete
I don't know when that will be

When will I be done?
Never. I hope
Because math is my treasure

Remember When

Emily Delbridge
Siegel High School, Grade 11

I remember when the world was green,
The grass was tall, the air was clean,
Sumptuous winds caressed bare skin,
Oh how I love to remember when.

Day by day and night by night,
We sent our dreams out into flight,
But all in all, we never knew:
A dream is a dream; it never comes true.

There were no bombs, no fiery skies,
No tempests raged in doleful eyes;
We knew no hate, nor greed, nor pain,
Just growth and gentle, cleansing rain.

And no one told us how to feel,
Or how to think or how to be;
We never knew the truth was lies,
Of hunger that makes children cry.

Once world of hope, once world for us:
Now shattered lives; the myth of trust.
So now I ache for those days again,
How sad it is to remember when.

He Helps Me Succeed

Amanda Neace
Smyrna West Alternative School, Grade 10

I follow my dreams,
And run from my nightmares,
I wake with a start,
Ready for a new day,
I follow those who help me succeed,
Hoping for the strength to one day lead,
I hit the ground hard when I tend to fall,
My fingers slip as I try to grasp the smooth wall,
Suddenly a strong hand reaches down from above,
He picks me up and shows me a smile of true love,
He kisses me gently and brushes away the dust,
He pushes me softly to do what I must,
My dreams come true,
My nightmares fade away,
Now I lead others without the slightest sway.

The Magic Pencil

Beau Waldron
Blackman Elementary School, Grade 5

Billy was a smart boy, but not a good student. He didn't like school and thought homework was a waste of time. He liked to try to find treasure in the neighborhood junkyard. And one afternoon he decided to go to the junkyard instead of studying for a test. While he was there, he saw something shining a few feet away. Billy took off running toward the shiny light and he tripped on something. While he was in the air he looked back and saw an old school desk and felt something hard and pointy hit his head. Much to his surprise, he had been hit by a pencil that flew from the desk.

Billy saw that the lead was silver, sharp, it had no eraser, and the words "use wisely" were on its side. He put it in his pocket and took it to school the next day. He was nervous as the test started . He didn't know any of the answers when he looked at the test. As he was writing his name, his pencil lead broke and he remembered the pencil he had put in his pocket.

When he grabbed it all the answers came to his head. Billy was the first one done with his test and made a 100%. He didn't tell anyone about his special pencil, but he continued to use it for all his work. He never studied but the pencil helped him make all A's. He was bragging about how smart he was.

A couple of weeks later, on the way to school, Billy's little brother saw the pencil and quietly took it. It was the day of the big six weeks exam. Of course, Billy had not studied. When he sat down to take his test he noticed that his pencil was not in his pocket. He had to guess on every answer and he failed.

Billy was embarrassed that he failed because he liked people thinking he was smart. Without his magic pencil he was left with only one thing to do. Study. Billy became a responsible student and learned that hard work pays off.

I'll Read Them All

Layton Miller
Buchanan Elementary School, Grade 5

The books! The books!
I'll read them all.
Of pirates, of seas,
They shall be mine.

Give me a book
Of good stories divine
Of dragons, of caves,
They shall be mine.

The books! The books!
I'll read them all
Of warriors, of planes,
They shall be mine.

Give me a book
Of good stories divine
Of witches, of rats,
They shall be mine.

Love

Cayla Spraggins
Stewarts Creek Middle School, Grade 7

True treasure is not found in pirate ships,
In chests of silver and gold.
True treasure isn't ruby rings
And jewels from long ago.
You don't need to use a treasure map
And find chests beneath the sea.
True treasure is simply the love
And joy found in you and me.

Guitar

Violet Kewley
Thurman Francis Arts Academy, Grade 2

I pick the strings
And out comes a song.
When everyone hears,
They sing along!

Dedication

Seth Dixon
Smyrna West Alternative School, Grade 9

You hold my secrets
My deepest thoughts
For no one else to see
The only one who knows my true identity
My mask is off
When I talk to you
Truth is all I speak
My fears come out
I'm at my most vulnerable point
Don't deceive me
Let no other eyes on thee
Your empty pages are filled with my life
I talk of the people that surround me
The bigots, the hypocrites, my lover that astounds me
All my thoughts convey to you
You keep me from going insane
Where would I be without the one
Who always listens to me
So I dedicate this page to you
As a token of appreciation
Ill never forget the time you spent
From keeping from ending this God's creation

A Treasure to Me

Marissa Hammond
Stewarts Creek Middle School, Grade 8

A treasure to me isn't a memory.
It is of my heart and soul.
My treasure is my God.
Each day I live is for Him.
Each breath I take is of Him.
I love Him, treasure Him, want Him, and need Him.
My treasure is my God.

Garden of a Child

Cassandra Handley
Blackman Elementary School, Grade 5

She looks around her and the world is filled with empty faces, hollow eyes
Demand allegiance from these narrow spaces, inside grows a secret flower
Thorny and wild
Risen from the long forgotten garden of a child

My Treasure

Jemina Leveque
Stewarts Creek Middle School, Grade 8

My treasure is sweet.
My treasure is fervent.
My treasure is flamboyant,
It makes me feel exuberant.
My treasure is intrepid and sometimes coy.
My treasure is versatile and sometimes full of turmoil.
My treasure is calm. My treasure is great.
You mess with my treasure; I'll become irate.
There are so many things my treasure could be but mostly I think my treasure is me.

Ring

Ashley Fleming
Blackman Elementary School, Grade 4

Ring
Hard, Gold
Shine, Sparkle, Glisten
I have a ring
Jewelry

Maine to Tennessee

Laci Cote
Blackman Elementary School, Grade 4

New places, new faces
From there to here
Glenburn, my hometown
Murfreesboro is where I live now.
Mad as I was, I moved
Away.
Never did I forget
Maine.
Still, I love Tennessee
My new home.

Lacy Is a Fat Cat

Harrison Stieber
Thurman Francis Arts Academy, Grade 2

Lacy is a cat
That is very, very fat.
Lying in the sun
Is what she does for fun.
Lacy is three,
And she loves me.
I love to hear her purr
And that is why I treasure her.

Green Frog

Kara Petty
Thurman Francis Arts Academy, Grade 4

There once was a little green frog.
Who liked to sit on a log.
He waited each day for a fly.
To eat quite quickly on the sly.

There once was a little green frog.
Who lived in a very deep bog.
He loved to sit in the sun.
Till the day was done.
There once was a little green frog.
Who liked to sleep under a log.
Till night came and passed.
Then, he would dash!

Nothing to Play

Jodi Chambers
Stewarts Creek Elementary School, Grade 4

One day
I was stuck in for the day
Nothing to play
Everybody was away

No one to play
I played with the dogs
I feed the frogs
But still no one to play

The Day I Became a Nerd

Legend Boun
Stewartsboro Elementary School, Grade 3

May 20, 2007 - The Test
"Today is the day for a vision test, " said Leon.
"I hope I pass the test," said Christopher.
Ding! The bell rang.

May 20, 2007 - It's Time
Today my teacher, Mrs. Miranda, called five people. One of those people was me. She said, "It's time for the vision test."
I got nervous after that as the five of us went to the room where we were to take the vision test.

May 20, 2007 – The Note
After I took my test, the doctor gave me a note. It said,
"Dear Parents of Leon,
Your son needs glasses.
　　　　Sincerely,
　　　　Mrs. Holiday"

May 20, 2007 – My Glasses
Tonight I gave the note to my mom and dad and they said, "This better not be about your grades!" As soon as they read it, my dad said, "We will get your glasses tomorrow."

May 23, 2007 – How It Happened
Today I went to school. People started calling me a nerd because of my glasses.
Christopher said, "Those people are calling you a nerd."
I said, " I know."
Then I went to the classroom. Next, people started to chuckle. Christopher told me to ignore them. I did what he said. I thought at least I have someone that respects me now.

Smooth as Ice

Austin Worrell
Smyrna West Alternative School, Grade 8

She is like glass,
so smooth and delicate.
Her heart is fragile,
so handle it with care.
Just because of her,
it is hard to breathe the air.
It is like stroking a snair,
as my heart begins to race.
Pace after pace,
I get closer and closer.
But when I see her,
I lose my composure.

France

Megan Dersu
LaVergne Middle School, Grade 8

"Bonjour ma Cherie, what can I get you on this fine evening?" The waiter said as I glanced over the selection of pastries. "The éclairs look delicious. I think I'll take two of those." I replied. As the waiter got the food I thought to myself, ahh.......France, what a place! France is the best place to live. Why you ask? The food is great, the fashion is extraordinary, and the sites are amazing. This is France!

Well, what can I say, I love food, and French food is delicious! France is home to the famous French bread, éclair, and, of course, the crème brulee. I thought to myself, if I lived in France I would eat these anytime I wanted, fresh from a French bakery. This is the first reason I want to live in France, the food.

Now, I'm not known for spending more than fifty dollars on a shopping trip, but I'm pretty sure living in France would break that habit! France is known for some of the best fashions in the world and some of the most extravagant shopping trips. I absolutely love French designers and clothes; this is another reason I want to live in France.

Sites! Sites! Sites! France is full of amazing sites. One such site would be the Eiffel Tower; another site would be Notre Dame. France is also known for its great shops and historical sites. France's list of sites is endless! This is another reason why France is the place to be.

In conclusion, France has got to be the best place to live. The food is delicious! The fashion will boggle your mind!! The sites are absolutely incredible!!! Tell me, where do you think is the best place to live?

U.S.A.
Thomas Garsnett
Thurman Francis Arts Academy, Grade 2

I LOVE my country because we are a FREE COUNTRY. Other countries have kings that make them go to churches that they don't want to go to. In our country, we have freedom of religion, and we can go to any church we want. In our country we have the freedom of speech and press. That means the government does not control what we speak and what we write. These freedoms are not free—we had to fight for our freedoms. Many soldiers have died for us to enjoy our FREEDOM.

My Treasure
Sean Dixon
Smyrna West Alternative School, Grade 8

Some people think a treasure is gold and silver.
No! A treasure is whatever you make it.
A treasure could be anything;
It could be someone special,
My treasure is in my heart.
You cannot follow a map and find it,
You cannot not dig it up,
This treasure has nothing to do with pirates
Or money.
My treasure is in my heart
Sealed up tight by a lock and chains
So no one will steal it.
My treasure is my life.

Talk to Me
Logan Coursey
Smyrna Middle School, Grade 7

Just because I'm short,
Don't think I'm stupid;
Don't make fun of me – be my friend.

Just because I'm short,
It doesn't mean I can't play football.
It doesn't mean I can't do good things.
It doesn't stop me from getting to high places.

Just because I'm short,
Still be my friend.
Can't wait 'till I get tall.

Just because I'm short – Please talk to me.

Treasure

Joey Meier
Oakland High School, Grade 12

Treasure is the crunch of pads amidst the sound of the band on a Friday night.
Treasure is the aroma of hot dogs and popcorn that fills the air.
Treasure is the sight of the ball sinking through the net in an overflowing gym.
Treasure is the sound of the coach's voice urging his men to victory.
Treasure is the crack of the bat on a spring night.
Treasure is the cheers from the crowd as the ball clears the fence and disappears
    into the night.
Treasure is the sound of the gun signaling the start of the race.
Treasure is the runner who crosses the line with sheer exhaustion on his face.
Treasure is not measured with wins or losses.
Treasure is measured in sweat and blood with pride, honor, and desire.
Treasure is the heart of a champion.

The Beast

James Kirk
Smyrna West Alternative School, Grade 7

Shiny little beast
Such a bad deed
To be greedy…greed

Nowhere else to go
Your feelings turn bold

Oh…Oh…Oh
…Gold

Treasure

Cheshire Rigler
Oakland High School, Grade 12

I am gold, diamonds, and priceless, sparkling jewels
I am family, friends, and a warm "welcome home"
I am the greedy desire of evil men
And the selfless desire of the righteous
I am a son, a daughter, a beloved spouse,
I am a destroyer of kingdoms, empires, and minds,
I am love,
I am insanity,
I am treasure!!!

15

Just Because I'm Short!

Katie B. Grisham
Smyrna Middle School, Grade 7

Just because I'm short,
Don't think I can't play basketball;
Don't think I can't shoot;
Don't think I can't dribble.
'Cause I can!

Just because I'm short,
Don't think I can't flip;
Don't think I can't do a handstand;
Don't think I can't do a cartwheel.
'Cause I can!

Just because I'm short,
Don't think I can't play volleyball;
Don't think I can't spike;
Don't think I can't hit the ball.
'Cause I can!

Just don't judge me
'cause I'm short.

Tsunami

James Jones
David Youree Elementary School, Grade 4

Rapid,
strong,
dangerous,
fast,
fierce,
bad,
huge,
outstanding,
amazing,
cool,
mad,
safari,
wavy,
and
scary.

Holding Up
Letress Orona
Smyrna Middle School, Grade 8

I had courage
Until you came
I had strength
Until you told me I was nothing
I believed in myself
Until you took that away from me
Now I see what you're all about
Girl after girl after girl
That's no way to treat a precious creation
If you love someone like you say you do
Then don't put that person down
It could lead to things you'll regret
Now I have courage
Now I have strength
Now I can finally believe in myself
Now you're gone….
I could care less….
Because you
You were nothing
Especially to me

Monster Trucks
Gage Howard
Blackman Elementary School, Grade 4

Monster trucks
Have big and wide wheels
Race around the track and destroy small cars
Are loud.

The Kingdom of Heaven
Jay Patton
Blackman Middle School, Grade 6

The Kingdom of Heaven is filled with His glory.
As I sing and dance to His story
Of when Jesus came and died for our sins
And wiped away the evil within
The Kingdom of Heaven is filled with His glory.

Treasures

Tashi McClain
Oakland High School, Grade 12

When one speaks of treasures one speaks of glitter and gold,
An abundance of wealth one wishes to behold.
Materialistic treasures are a specious treasure
Compared to love that lasts forever.
Love will never tarnish or rust with age
Or fly away like a bird in a cage.
The greatest treasures in life are
The loving moments we share
With loved ones who honestly care.

Life from A to Z

Ayinde Bakari
Blackman Middle School, Grade 6

Avoid negative energy
Believe in yourself
Consider the possibilities
Do the right thing
Experience life
Fulfill your dreams
Giving all you can
Has fun
Introduce new things
Just do your best
Keep out negative people
Let go of all anger
Make your dreams happen
Never let people say you can't
Only look to the future
Practice being a better person
Question all your problems
Remember your dreams
Stop blaming yourself
Think positively
Understand all your problems
Visualize all good things
Want something; go after it
'Xcel in life
You are special just the way you are
Zero in on all your dreams

Lion King
Christian Copeland, Brice Britton, Maria Quaintance
David Youree Elementary School, Grade 4

Lion
Eats meat daily
Females hunt while males
Feed
King of beasts watching over
The pride
Lion King

About the Treasure
Olivia Perry
Blackman Elementary School, Grade 1

One day I was playing outsid and I fowned a treasur. I put it in my closet and I invitid my frined over to see it. The end.

My Treasures
Michaela Cain
Blackman Middle School, Grade 7

Some people's treasure is money.
Some people's treasure is fame,
but the treasures that I carry are quite plain.
They are
family,
love,
and happiness!

My Treasure!
Mitchell Reed
Blackman Elementary School, Grade 1

My treasure was a juoul and it is speshol to Me.

My Treasures
Josie Wornstaff
Blackman Elementary School, Grade 1

My puppy is my treasure and I love him so much!

My Dream

Emily Elizabeth Ericson
Blackman Middle School, Grade 8

I dream of becoming a writer as my career,
I'll be a writer for sixty more years.
I have many stories in my brain.
I hope my dream won't go down the drain.
I write suspense that will make you jump with fright!
I have thirty stories going through my head that I will soon write.
My dream is to be an author forever.
You will stop me never.

My Most Valuable Treasure

Lauren Zachary
Rockvale Elementary School, Grade 3

My most valuable treasure is my doll Elmo. He is one of my friends. I got him when I was just six months old, and I've slept with him ever since. This year he is eight years old and so am I. It is good to be friends with Elmo.

My Dog Pickles

Marian Leonard
Thurman Francis Arts Academy, Grade 5

I love my dog Pickles
she's very special to me.
She makes me laugh and giggle
As she chases squirrels up the trees.

She sleeps with me at night
Then wakes me up in the morning
She's very, very fun
Although she can be boring.

I hate it when she gets into trouble,
She has to go outside for the day.
But that just gives me a reason
To go outside to run and play.

The cat scratches her a lot
It makes her cry and whimper.
She hops and skips when I get home,
We should have named her skipper!

Music

Mary-Grace Williams
Homer Pittard Campus School, Grade 5

The love I treasure for music is priceless. The notes flowing through my mind. I feel like I'm on top of the world when I sing. Like I've accomplished something new. I treasure music, because it's been in my family for generations, and I'm always caught in the notes. It is like they're flying through the sky.

Dream

Virginia Tipps
Homer Pittard Campus School, Grade 5

Dream, that's a strong word. What it means to me is to have hope and faith. To fulfill your dream is a big accomplishment. My dream is to be a better person, to help and be helped by people that are close to me and to people who aren't.

I think everyone needs to have a dream or something to strive for. Dream can mean different things, it can mean what you do when you're asleep (in bed or in class), or it can mean to have something to work and sometimes wish for. So keep your dream alive in your heart and don't let anyone tell you what to dream for. I will forever treasure my dreams.

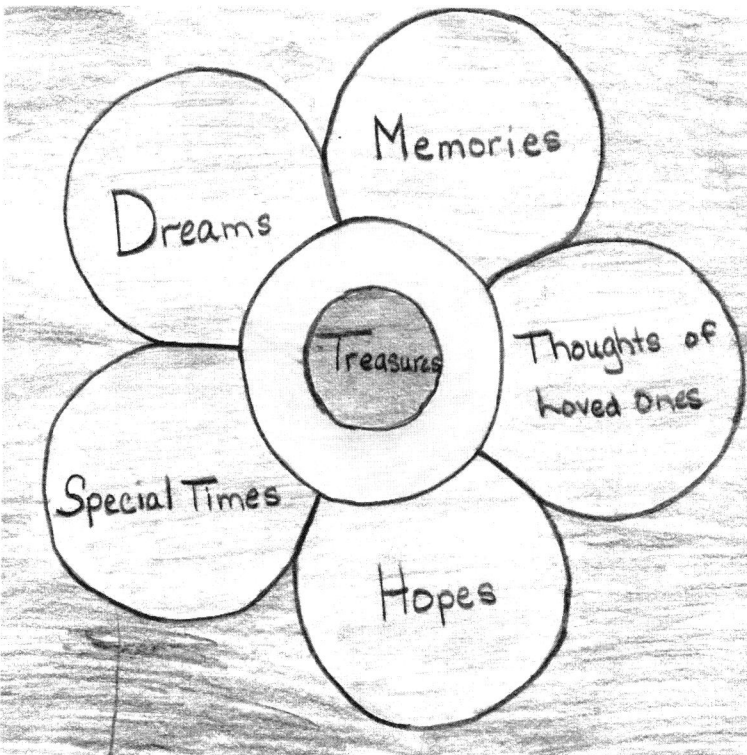

Rachel Lynch, Eagleville School, Grade 6

21

Stories

Julia Walsh
Homer Pittard Campus School, Grade 5

They make me laugh
They make me cry
They make me feel
So happy inside

Stories are my bread and
Butter; they make me feel
So full

They take me on adventures
They take me to the past
They fill my head with knowledge
And my heart with courage, too

They give me secrets,
They give me strength
They make me wonder,
Make me think,
Make me remember
Make me forget

So next time you listen
To a story, just close your eyes
And forget your problems and
Your worries

Just fall into a trance of
Listening and learning
From the story that's at hand.

Stories are my treasure they're
Very dear to me
They never fade they never
Go they're always with me
Wherever I go.

My Kittens

Jason Raines
Wilson Elementary School, Kindergarten

I have four kittens and one is really special because he has three legs. They sleep in my bed with me and I play fetch with them.

My Special Kitty

Savannah Young
Wilson Elementary School, Grade 2

One day a soft, fluffy, white cat showed up on my front porch. I asked my mom if I could keep her and she said Yes! I named her Snowflake. She was my first pet. I give her milk and food every morning. I like when she cuddles with me. She is my special treasure because I love her and she loves me!

The Creek

Brooklynne Bell
Blackman Middle School, Grade 8

As I sit passively in the backseat of my car, I glance out the window and catch, by chance, a small path meandering through the trees, dodging rocks and roots alike. The simple sight stirs a memory in me, hidden behind more recent concerns of homework and housework. I remember the Creek and am moved back in time.

After a quick shout to my mother, my friend Devin and I dash to the entrance of the Creek, only about a hundred yards away at the end of the cul-de-sac. Our hearts beat much more quickly, excitement shoving adrenaline through our systems and smiles onto our faces. We stop and exchange a wry glance. "Are you thinking what I'm thinking?" I asks Devin, a roguish smile making its silent way up my cheeks. She nods. We dash away and run to the other entrance, where a dirty road cuts the Creek in half. We turn right and look down, facing three large, silver tunnels below our feet, below the road. I nudge Devin. "You go first." She shrugs, as if it were no difficult task at all, then makes her descent to the bottom of the six foot drop between the top of the tunnels and the block of cement supporting them. After a few minutes, she looks up at me and grins, rubbing the only scrape on her elbow. She motions for me to follow her, but I shake my head fearfully. I dart to the other, much simpler entrance and duck to elude the low tree branches. I smile, content with my surroundings and with the knowledge that I am unscathed, but also dissatisfied that I hold no battle scars. Yet.

The Creek, green, gorgeous, and wet, was a spacious area containing picturesque evergreen and deciduous trees surrounding living room-sized plains of rocks, puddles, and ponds. There was a natural platform of rock that made a pathway into the heart of the Creek. As a young child, I would always turn my feet and discover, once again, a woodsier area with a fallen tree that one could never manage to avoid tripping over. Further along the pathway lay a beautiful area with cacti, more rocks, and a slow-moving stream swirling lazily around the last few boulders sticking up out of the greenish water.

Mystical beings heavily populated the Creek. The magical quality of the green wilderness was so beautiful, so fresh, so *wild* that we couldn't help but imagine any number of enchanted creatures: Fairies whispered mysterious secrets in our ears, and wood nymphs peeked timidly out from behind trees; unicorns cantered past our vision while the wind blew in our faces, wheezing of the sights it had seen. Once a dragon even visited our little enchanted corner of the world, catching everything on fire as mermaids sprayed water on the intangible inferno until the great winged lizard tired of us and left.

The last time I visited the Creek was this past April, about a year and a half after we moved away from the house by the Creek. I had completely lost touch with Devin and my other neighborhood friends. My sister said to me, "Hey, I'm going to the Creek. Want to come?" I agreed, and we drove to our old neighborhood, only twenty minutes away. What I saw completely and overwhelmingly disturbed me. I could effortlessly climb down the tunnel to the ground. I followed my sister to the deeper clearing, easily stepping over the fallen tree. The whole place just seemed . . . smaller, somehow. Less significant. In the deeper clearing, I looked around and gasped. Graffiti covered the rocks where I had conversed with the mermaids. As I stepped through the once waist-high grass, something caught my shoe. It seemed to be the last hope of a desperate fairy, calling me to assist the place, but as I examined closer, I saw that it was just a long piece of withered brown grass, coincidentally catching my sock, by no means a fairy. I choked back a sob. Now as I drive away, I hit upon a realization, my heart heavy. Some things can't help but change.

Love
Joe Winkler
Rockvale Elementary School, Grade 7

Love....
Love is like a bird on its first flight
Like a candle sharing its light
Love is a newborn flame
Like a baby gaining its name
Love is kind and leads your fate
With it you create and without it you hate.
Love creates freedom, for one and all
If there were no love this world would surely fall.

Joy

Corrine Wheeler
Rockvale Elementary School, Grade 7

Joy, the twinkle in a child's eye
The purring kitten of your heart
The angel that breathes life into your soul
And the wish you make upon a star
Joy is the person swinging you by your feet
And carrying you up above the highest mountain
Joy is the cloud you float on, what number is it again?
A never ending rainbow that flows into your mind.
Joy is a butterfly first spreading its wings
A duckling learning to swim
And the strength it takes to never give in
In the end joy is joy in itself
A circle that starts and hopefully never ends.

Treasures

Maggie Lou Warren
McFadden School of Excellence, Grade 2

My treasure was the tooth I lost.

I was so happy when I lost it that I gave it to the Tooth Fairy.

She gave me two dollars.

Losing a tooth is fantastic!

I sure hope the Tooth Fairy will treasure my tooth.

The Choice

Monique Lovelady
Oakland High School, Grade 11

You can believe in yourself and do the best you can.
You can follow your heart and take a stand.
Or you can give up easily and be filled with tears.
And have to one day look back on your fears.
You can face the fact that life isn't fair,
And don't expect anyone to care.
Or you can whine, and yell and complain,
And feel so hurt when you see life isn't a game.
You can do whatever you can to make your dreams come true,
Or you can keep on wishing and dreaming,
The choice is up to you.

My Horse Whisper

Stormie Cook
Lascassas Elementary School, Grade 4

When I was three years old, I took riding lessons and my daddy bought me a horse. My horses's name is Whisper. She is white and black and has blue eyes. My parents say she looks like me. The vet says that this is called glass eyes. She is very nice, and she means the world to me.

Whisper and I do contests and shows together. Whisper came to my house for my birthday one year. I had sixteen of my closest friends come to my party. That was one of my favorite birthdays ever. Whisper and I did an egg hunt together one Easter. She wore a pretty Easter bonnet. My mom had made it for her.

All of my friends that I have taken to meet Whisper love her. She likes it when I bring her carrots. She enjoys it when my mom and I give her a bath and brush her. We clean her hooves.

About two years ago, Whisper had a baby girl named Maisy. My granddaddy and mom bred Whisper with a miniature horse. Maisy is my little sister's pony. She loves her, too. Whisper is a very good mommy.

Whisper now lives on my granddaddy's farm in Readyville with Maisy. My family and I love her very much.

Things I Treasure

Shawn Culp
Christiana Elementary School, Grade 5

Most people treasure…
Silver, jewels, or gold
But behold, I don't treasure gold

I treasure my family
I'm glad to have a mom and dad
They always care for me
They rarely make me mad
They are part of my family tree

I have a girlfriend
I hope we'll never end
I also have a best friend
Our weirdness will always blend

I have an electric guitar
That I've learned so far
I love Jesus
He always loves us
That's just a start
Of the things I treasure

A Little Magic

Maia Lewis
Holloway High School, Grade 10

A forest. Soft, still, and beckoning. A hint of magic. Secret, haunting, and whispering. I creep forward and hear the faint tinkling of bells and laughter. I peer through the bushes and I am there.

Acorn goblets, toadstool seats, a stone table, vast and bountiful. Elderberry wines, honeysuckle juice, chutes, roots, and petals. Berries and fruits of all kinds known to man, and some that remain undiscovered. Leaf plates piled high with wild rice and pumpkin pie, Dancing and laughter, a band's merry hum. Spider silk gowns and armor made from pinecones. A queen, fairer than all, smiles at the moon. I steal away, and that cheery music will stay in my mind forever.

Solitude

Loren Lester
Oakland High School, Grade 11

Lost in shadows of the night
With only the moon as my light.
I wander the shrouding darkness
With only my thoughts of loneliness.

I ponder the meaning of solitude.
And with each passing day
Accept it with more gratitude.
How much of a treasure it truly is
To rely on oneself as much as this.

I continue on through the trees
Accompanied only by a soft breeze.
I then came to a place I know by heart
The place where you promised me
We would never be apart.

And I stand there and wonder,
With my face to the skies.
How solitude is truly a treasure,
As the tears fall from my eyes.

Treasures

Hank Becker
Siegel Middle School, Grade 6

Around the world people look for gold
>They start when they're young and finish when old.

Pirates plunder what others have gotten
>People don't like them; they think they are rotten.

Big shiny jewels people like to wear
>They stick them on fingers and put them in hair.

Stocks and bonds and tons of cash
>What people love most is having a stash.

People put paintings up on their walls
>They show them off to friends that call.

These things are stuff that anyone can get
>They're not worth a lot, on that we can bet.

Real treasure of life: God, family, and friends
>Just follow your heart and look within.

The Ostracized Faceless

Mahalia Paraiso
Riverdale High School, Grade 11

Solace, solitude
Put me under lock and key
No one knows my name anyway
My room is a safe
Only one person can free me
All are too distracted by the mirrors
Constantly, stupidly staring at themselves
Meanwhile, I'm blind and slowly die
I lie behind the mirror
And only one person bothers to look for me
Good thing I don't realize it
Or I might go mad
Put me under lock and key
No one knows my name anyway

Every Day

Kylie Putnal
Siegel High School, Grade 9

Every day is a gift
24 more hours of life
Every day is a memory
of our accomplishments and strife
Every day is a blessing
a privilege to us all
Every day is another chance
for us to stand when we fall
Every day is a winding road
leading to somewhere unknown
Every day is a new experience
an unsteady stepping stone
Every day is another chapter
in our never-ending story
Every day is another step
in our life-long journey
Every day is an adventure
a chance to rediscover the world
Every day is an opportunity
for us to change the world

Terms of Silence

Kelcey Evans
Oakland High School, Grade 11

Misused words.
Unspoken pain.
Love gone wrong.
Repeating shame.
Thoughts provoked.
Actions untaken.
A downward spiral.
Life gone to shame.
What more to do?
Shall we sit and wait?
Watch life go to waste,
and let love make mistakes.
Or shall we take a stand;
Make life right again?
So that we may laugh,
live, and love till our
very end.

A Brighter Day

Kayla Van Winkle
Oakland High School, Grade 11

When things
Aren't going
The way you would like them to,
Don't turn your back even though it is the easiest thing to do.

When everything seems to be going wrong,
And you feel like everyone and everything is helping the bad times along,
Do not give up your fight.
Do not go astray.
Because if you make it through the night,
Tomorrow is a brighter day.

When the world is crumbling down on you,
And you feel there is nothing you can do.
When every last one of your dreams has fallen to your feet,
And your head hangs down in defeat

Do not give up your fight.
Do not go astray.
Because if you make it through the night,
Tomorrow is a brighter day.

For if you give up your fight,
If you go astray,
Then the night was too long, and it took from your light.
Now, tomorrow may never come your way.
A brighter day may never come your way.

So don't give up your fight.
You can make it through the night.
To see a brighter day
Come your way.

My Pocket

MaryGrace Bouldin
Homer Pittard Campus School, Grade 3

In my pocket you can find…
A pair of glasses, an old valentine.

A polka-dot pencil, a rubber band,
My brother's action figure, a plastic hand.

A sheet of stars, a teddy bear,
Last week's schedule, a piece of hair.

A banana peel (from last year),
A picture of a blue sea pier.

An ink stain, and the pen it came out of,
And lots of things I have not said above.

My sweat-shirt pocket I should not tell,
The last person I told just suddenly fell!

Poem

Ryan Baxter
Thurman Francis Arts Academy, Grade 6

These are items that I treasure,
glittering gems and eagle feathers.
These wonders of the natural world,
can disappear with all that's pearled.
Everything can wash away
in the length of a single day.
All gone in a matter of time,
not brought back with every dime.
Let the little children shout,
and let every voice cry out.
Don't let your words be fake,
If you speak true, a difference you'll make.

The Fire of Missions

Savannah Shepherd
Smyrna High School, Grade 9

In remembrance of all those whose lives were uprooted by Katrina and my youth
group's trip for disaster relief summer of 2006.

I went to Mississippi and walked its coast
Left in ruins like a parasite's host
I saw the destruction and sorrow of the land
Left like that by Katrina's hand
In the ghost of a vision left to rot
I found eight inch glass as if shattered by a gunshot
But these were not what struck me the most:
The wind, the waves on the shattered coast
But a saucer without a chip or a crack
Lying among the eight inches of glass
Now it is time for a new chapter to be written
I'm going to Mexico so the devil's work will be smitten
There we are taking the word of God
So one day everyone will bow and head will nod
By the witness of our hearts and Christ's sacrifice
Through the prejudice and hate God's love will slice
I want to come back with my heart in a new place
But his fire still burning, me still in the race
Some people have a heart for the black or the white
But my vision Lord is for all in sight
So send me Lord into the nations
To take your love to all the races
That they now may know your name
And have a heart just the same.

My Treasures

Josh Little
Christiana Elementary School, Grade 5

T is for the trips I take.
R is for the rights I have.
E is for the experiences I have with my family.
A is for my aunts that are special to me.
S is for my brother's spirit.
U is for my uncles that love me.
R is for my Grandpa Richard.
E is for the excitement I have when I'm around my friends.

Our Pride

Abby Duke
Christiana Middle School, Grade 8

The red, white, and blue flag spread over the casket
The sense of freedom
The anthem resonating through the dense air
The sadness of the family and friends
The pride of the soldiers
Patriotism is one of our greatest treasures

A Gentle Touch

Olivia Branscomb
Oakland High School, Grade 9

A gentle touch
A glimpse of fear
A thought of hope
I reached for her hand
Wrinkled and old
Her face shown with joy
All she said was "thanks"
And walked away

One Window

Dalton Carter
Christiana Middle School, Grade 8

One window is all I need
To make a change in someone's life
For the health of everyone in the world around
To see people for who they are
To keep my feet on the ground
To see the "X" that marks the spot
And to find the treasure buried within

My Treasure Chest

Caroline Daws
Siegel High School, Grade 9

I wonder where my treasures lie.
Is it the warmth in a summer's day,
or the beauty in a flake of snow?
Is it the rippling of a bride's gown,
or the look in her father's eyes when he gives her away?

Is it the bright smile of a friend
whose love can brighten
even the worst of days?
Or the sound of rolling thunder
from a cloud growing every moment darker?

Is it in the hope of a child
Or a mother's touch, so gentle and loving?
Is it the last resonating tone of a symphony
when one wishes it would never cease,
so locks it away in the mind and throws away the keys?

I wonder where my treasures lie?
Are they in the past, the future,
do they exist in time?
Are they bound by our limits,
our fears, our wants?
Or do they soar in a place indescribable, extravagant,
untouched by the world?

Beautiful Butterflies

Tierra Parker
Smyrna Primary School, Grade 5

Colorful butterflies in the air,
As we walk past,
Like a rainbow in the sky,
Around they go,
See you tomorrow.

Not Only Them...

Jocie Hofstra
Oakland High School, Grade 9

To take what you could give away
To keep what you could share
Leave it alone
All for you
All for me
Accept the rejection
I promise
To them it's fair
It may hurt now
Tomorrow too?
To them it will matter
I've watched many a victim fall
Held at arms length
Not only them...
But us all.

The Day My Cousin Came Home from Iraq

Matthew Cook
Smyrna Primary School, Grade 5

It's November 11th and the guns fire and the flags fly. Our soldiers arrive in their uniforms, tears were falling, people were leaping into the sky, people were hollering, and everywhere you looked there were hugs. When I walked around to find my cousin, my eyes filled with water and started raining tears of joy. When I found my cousin, it was like a Christmas present that had come true. I ran toward him and bound into his arms and wrapped my arms around him with a firm grip. I didn't let go until he said, "You are killing me." That is when I released my arms and let him go. I fell to the ground and backed up so that the next person did not run over me. Then, the next person gives him an enormous hug. Finally, we walk to the car and put his stuff up while he returns his weapons. We head home for him to rest. He says that it feels good to be home and not hearing the sounds of gunfire every second. He loves being with his family. Please pray for the troops that are still there and their families. They may not be coming home and their families will not be able to experience the joy I felt that day.

Tireless in Tennessee

Brian Allen
Siegel High School, Grade 9

There once was a fearful man,
Who was single with no life plan.
He could not sleep in the eerie night;
All he could do was sit in bed and write.

His creepy, dilapidated house was eighty years old,
It was drafty so the nights were uncomfortably cold,
As darkness set in, the wooden floors began to creak
Thoughts of another sleepless night made him shriek.

In anticipation of the night,
With no neighbors in sight,
His imagination turned his irrational fear
Into a reality that only he could hear.

The man's passion and talent to write
Gave him freedom from his fright.
It channeled his imagination to his verse
Instead of the senseless fear of the looming curse.

His urge to write took the fear away.
He focused on his work 'til the break of day.
As the dawn replaced the night
Sleep was no longer a fight.

No More Wars

Blake Howland
Lascassas Elementary School, Grade 4

I have a dream that there will be no more wars in the world. People would be happier.
Families would not be sad because they are not separated. That's why there should be
no more wars.

Saw You
Destiny Fathera
Siegel High School, Grade 9

I saw you in the hailstorm
The thunder and the rain,
I saw you in the sunshine
And still you looked the same,
I saw you when you did
What you thought you'd never do,
When I closed that open door
And you missed the window to crawl through,
I saw you when you cried
And your tears hit the ground,
When you discovered the joy
You thought couldn't be found,
I saw you fall down the mountain
And climb up again,
When I whispered in the dark
This is your battle to win,
I saw you when you denied me
And when you came to the truth,
I saw you when you loved me
When you gave me all of you

My Pet Rocky
Andrew Dodge
Blackman Elementary School, Grade 3

One of the things I treasure is my pet guinea pig Rocky. Rocky is very cute and has black fur on her body. Around her nose she is white. She always runs around in her cage. She loves to eat lettuce and carrots. When I let her play in her castle maze, she always runs for cover inside the castle. A few months ago we found out she is a girl. She also likes to chew on a lot of things. She is a treasure to me.

Priceless Treasure

Gabi Gumucio
Stewarts Creek Middle School, Grade 6

5000 miles
10,000 waves
Knowing I'm finally there at Treasure Caves

Seeing the chest I have been traveling to see
Wondering what's inside
What will it be?

Finally being able to open it up
Hoping that it will be so full of jewels and gold
That it will erupt.

Instead it erupted with all the treasures I never acknowledge I already have.
Seeing pictures of aunts, uncles, cousins, sister, brothers, moms, dads, and even friends, too.
Now knowing these are the most important treasures to both me and you.

Treasures in Heaven

Kaitlyn Palmer
Lascassas Elementary School, Grade 6

When I think of treasures, I think of Matthew 6:19-21. "Do not store up for yourselves treasures on earth, where moth and rust destroy, and where thieves break in and steal. But store up for yourselves treasures in Heaven where moth and rust do not destroy and where thieves do not break in and steal. For where your treasure is, there your heart will be also." This verse to me means you don't need to be worried about all your possessions. After our house was broken into recently, I realized how unimportant our things are here on earth. They can always be replaced. It doesn't matter what was taken from our home. What matters the most is that we still have each other and we know God will take care of us as long as we trust in Him.

My Picture

Shelby Stroud
Smyrna High School, Grade 11

Words mean nothing
Unless you can feel them,
Your mouth speaks the words
Your heart knows how to use them.

Sometimes I say words
I hope you know I don't mean.
I don't always listen to my heart
And I hope you do forgive me.

Every time you say
Anything to me
It's more than just words
Love is what I see.

You already knew these things
Now I can know them, too.
That's why every time I think of love
I can't help but picture you.

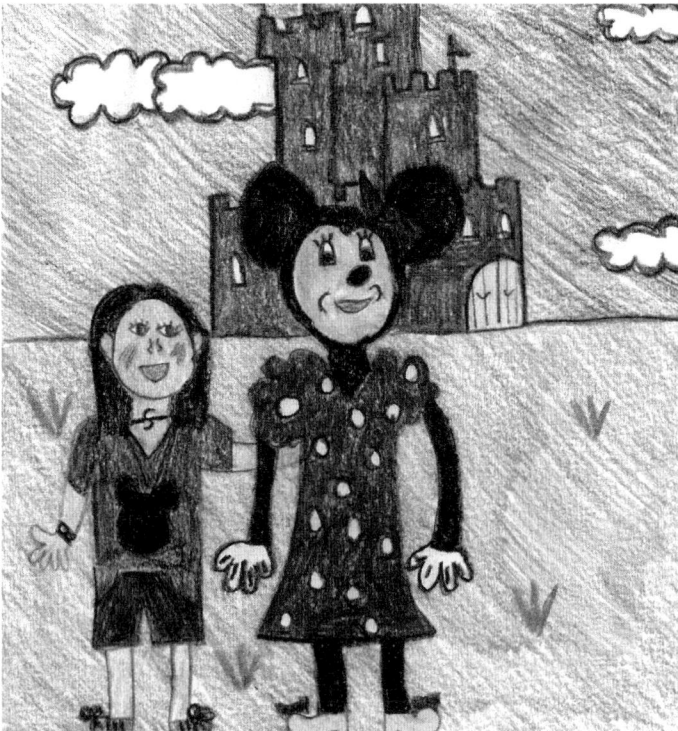

Savannah Berry, McFadden School of Excellence, Grade 5

What Unites Us

Ashli Williams
Siegel High School, Grade 9

What could be solid darkness
Is filled with city lights.
Beauty is the sharpness
Of New York City nights.
And through the misting rain,
People rush to urban sights
While one girl on a train
Looks up at all those lights.
She knows it in her heart;
It is her treasure in her life.
She could not spend one night apart
From New York City sights.

One thousand miles away
The sun is going down.
A man observes a field of hay,
His farm's colors – green and brown.
There is no motion or sound for miles.
He has not a thing to say.
Grass and food and crops in piles
City chaos is his dismay
And although they are worlds apart,
This man too has found his treasure.
The silent dusk warms his heart
Life in the country is his pleasure.

Many different lives are led
Across the world as we know it.
Of growing wheat and grain for bread,
Having something to show for it.
Of Saturday nights at the symphony hall,
Glamour and culture, having it all.
Of an entire life searching for skill,
A basketball game, victory's buzzing trill.
Of university and successful inquisition,
Career and having paramount position.
Of a hard day's work, rewarding and sweet,
Loving each day, in the cold or the heat.
We are all however united by a common desire
Like a droplet makes rain, or a flame makes a fire
It stands so true for each of us, for all
That perfect bliss is having someone come when we call.

Our treasures come from living styles, we say
From cows or sports, from college or Broadway
But the treasures of love are far too universal
To be compared to coaching or to orchestra rehearsal.

That girl watching the world from New York City
Was on the train to her niece's birthday party.
That man in the field of his successful farm
Was taking care of his son, who had broken his arm.
A woman in a hidden corner of that symphony hall
Had married the concertmaster just that past fall.
That professional basketball player from Montana
Had left a daughter at home he missed named Savannah.
That man working hard at university needed to know
How to cure his mother's schizophrenia before she would go.
As that man tasted the sweat from his day's hard aggression
He was working to pay for his fiancé's prized possession.
We all believe that we are so different from each other
But we all understand what we all are working for.
For our uncle, girlfriend, husband, mother, and brother
Nothing really seems like such a chore.
We have this is common, and it is forever true
Our greatest treasure is to hear someone say, "I love you."

Do YOU Really See?

Lace' Tomlinson
Smyrna High School, Grade 11

Through the life of children
we see
Through the cry of the nation
we hear
Through the love of a family
we feel
We see what we want to see
We listen to what we want to hear
But what we feel cannot be controlled
just felt, just listen
just see

My Treasured Doll

McKenzie Tatum
Rock Springs Middle School, Grade 6

On Christmas Eve two years ago, I got my second American Girl doll, Anna Paige Tatum. She is very special to me because she gives me comfort when I'm feeling down. When I let my imagination run wild, it seems as if she's there and really talking to me.

I love playing teacher. Of course, Anna is always there being an intelligent student. She also has classmates, Eliza and Marisol, who are also American Girls. Sometimes I do the girls' hair and dress them up. Then we do a fashion show, which Anna loves.

Anna's quite the traveler. She and I have been many places together. Her favorite trip was to the American Girl store in Chicago, where she met her little sister Marisol. She's been many different places such as Disney World, St. Louis, and on lots of visits to our grandparents' house.

You could definitely say Anna's my treasure. Anna's very pretty and she looks a lot like me. I don't even know what I would do without her.

I always have a great time playing with Anna: I know she has a wonderful time on vacations. If she could talk, she would say, "I love you, Mommy!" Anna is my treasure!

The Treasure of My Heart

Laci Gibbs
Smyrna High School, Grade 12

I embarked on a journey,
The journey of life,
To find a treasure
Of the fair heart of mine.
I discovered a chest,
Full of diamonds and gold.
I knew it would only last
Until I grew old.
I wanted something valuable
But more than diamonds and gold
Something less tangible
To have and to hold.
For worldly treasures
Will wither away
Along with their pleasures
Lasting less than a day.
I want to remember
And cherish forever

My heart's truest treasure
That I have yet to discover.
My footsteps are guided
By a beautiful map.
The straight pathway is lighted
To where my treasure is.
Where "X" marked the spot
There a note lay:
"The treasure of life is not gold
But the life that you've made."
The treasure of my heart,
I found along the way.
Those precious moments
With my dear family.

The White Morning

Sabrina Spicer
Stewarts Creek Elementary School, Grade 5

I went outside, the cold wind hit my face
I go back inside and start to pace
What to do on my fabulous snowy day
I call my friends to see if they can play
They can. That's great! I grab my coat
They grab toys and a plastic boat
We meet in the dim, morning light
We build a snowman flying a kite
Soon we make a sea of snow
And a sailor with a bow
Then mom calls; it's time to go in
We take off our scarves and go to the den
She serves use hot coco and cookies with milk
And we cover ourselves with a blanket of silk
As Mittens our cat jumps to see if we can play
She suddenly pulls the cover away
Then my friends off to bed
Soon will come the man in red!

The Coming Weather

Sabrina Spicer and Samantha Blankenship
Stewarts Creek Elementary School, Grade 5

As I stepped outside I saw a mural of oranges, yellows, and reds
Falling from the once lively trees of the orchard were leaves of dead
They looked as if they were frowning in sorrow
But as you know they may be gone tomorrow
They fell as gently as feathers
This all part of the coming weather

Buried Treasure

Allison Thomas
Siegel High School, Grade 10

I buried my heart
a long time ago.
I buried it in a spot
that no one did know.

I hid the key
somewhere so deep,
the finder will win
my soul to keep.

I forgot the place
I hid the key.
If someone would please
find it for me?

You followed the clues
 that led to my key.
You've won my heart
and gave yours to me.

You found the treasure
I buried so long ago.
You dug up my heart
from the spot no one did know.

You found my buried treasure.

Summer

Aaron Kuhn
McFadden School of Excellence, Grade 5

Summer is so much fun,
Even when you are in the hot sun.

You can get a tan,
But it feels like you are a hot pan.

Summer is so cool,
It's fun to get in the pool.

Summer is my favorite time of year,
We can play all day because the skies are so clear.

It is such fun to catch fireflies at night,
They are so easy to see because of their tail light.

We cookout and stay up late,
Hotdogs and hamburgers fill my plate.

At night when I close my eyes,
I look forward to another day of surprise.

Treasures

Quinton Lasko
Siegel Middle School, Grade 7

Treasures are important things
A treasure can be a word
That causes happiness
A treasure can be a person
That spreads joy to everyone around him or her
A treasure can be an item
That makes you express an emotion
Treasures are important things

A Wolf's Life

Katie Stueckle
Rock Springs Elementary School, Grade 4

Ow, ow, awooooo! Yes, I'm a wolf. If you like stories about cute chipmunks, look elsewhere. This story is not cute. Well, let's get to the point.

My name is Cloudberry. I have a twin called Midnight. I'm older by six minutes, but we're both eight years old. Our lives have been full of hardships. Anyway, this is what we look like: I am a white wolf with yellow eyes, and Midnight is a black wolf with brown eyes. Midnight gets annoying, so sometimes I have to toss her around. This is the story of our lives.

Our mother died giving birth to Midnight with our brother still inside her. Three months later, a moose struck our father dead. Five years later, hunters took our brave pack. Midnight and I were taken in small metal dens to a huge white den. Then…horror! I saw our pack's furs hanging on the wall! I struggled so frantically that my cage toppled into Midnight's and the doors burst open! We flew outside and didn't stop running until we got to our den. There we came to an abrupt halt, because at our den was a grizzly sow feeding her cubs our store of meat! Midnight whimpered and stuck her tail between her legs. We turned tail and ran.

Suddenly, a column of boiling water and steam shot up under Midnight's left forepaw and the tip of my tail. We yelped in pain and I realized that we'd run into a geyser field! We limped as fast as we could to a compact and cozy cave. There we nursed our scalded wounds. The land of Yellowstone is very dangerous!

The next morning we woke up with fevers. Our pack (before they died) had told us about the sulfur-water that chased away fever. I loped along behind Midnight, following the faint sulfur scent. Suddenly, Midnight disappeared! Then she reappeared, a bedraggled, shiny-eyed mass of fur. She panted to tell me that this was sulfur-water! Sploosh! I leapt into the hot water and drank gratefully. Soon our fevers had gone, and we went hunting. Almost immediately, I spotted a small elk herd and recognized it as the weak Lamara valley herd. I glimpsed a recently-dead elk carcass and descended upon it to eat. Midnight followed. Hunger satisfied, we went back to our cave. That day we also explored part of our territory. Over the course of the next week, we set boundaries and explored the rest of our territory. There were many geysers and enchanting hot pools.

Ever since all that happened, Midnight and I have lived in our cave, as old-age wolves. We tell stories to the young ones. We are called "The Tellers." We are the honored wolf elders.

Now you have heard our story.

Treasures

Brooke Routh
Blackman Elementary School, Grade 4

Gold is for me. Gold is for you.
Gold is old. Gold is new.
Gold is shiny but can't be blue
Gold is valuable can this be true.
If I find some, I'll share with you.

Treasures

Rachel Bazzell
Christiana Elementary School, Grade 5

I treasure many things. I treasure my friends, family, pets, and music. I treasure my friends and family because no matter how big of a fight we get in or how mad we get at each other they still love me. They are always there for me.

I treasure music the most because I can play it and listen to it. Music makes me feel better when I am mad, sad, or even confused. There is always a song that makes it better.

Angel

Shellie Anderson
Eagleville School, Grade 5

Pink, blue, and white
Sadness and happiness
I remember someone special.

In a little red box
Under my bed
Only take it out on Christmas
The day I can remember him.

If anything happened
To my little angel
I could still see it
In my heart
My little angel.

Treasures Poem

Weston Wax
Siegel High School, Grade 12

A treasure is a piece of one's heart,
Something that's priceless, eternal, and sacred.
It may be a precious heirloom, a pair of jeans bought at Wal-mart,
A boy's dug up collections of coke cans stashed in his tree house, or a girl's hallowed
love letter kept in a box underneath her bed.

A treasure is a poison to one's heart.
An item at an auction that's turned the buyer's blood green with greed,
And turned his heart to stone before the biddings have commenced.
The one obsession that demands the purchaser takes no heed.

A treasure is an antidote to one's heart,
Giving meaning where emptiness once was;
A glimmer of hope where despair had oppressed;
A flicker of sunshine where the clouds had blanketed over before;
A passion in place of contentment;
And an excitement instead of the mundane.

A treasure could be anything you make it,
But no matter what, the common denominator of a treasure's equation is the heart.
Be it a pure and holy relic or a wretched awful bit.
Deep inside the chest of someone is where the meaning of a treasure starts.

In Christ's Love

Dreams

Angelique Sloan
Central Middle School, Grade 8

Dreams go fast and far these days
They go by rocket thrust
Dreams can be very old these days
Or very new
They need no special charts
They need not any fuel
It seems only one rule
Applies to all our dreams
They will not fly
Except in open sky
A fenced in dream will die.

49

Treasures

Emily Lupoli
Siegel High School, Grade 12

A treasure can be many things,
A treasure can be small,
A treasure can be bracelets or rings,
A treasure can be anything at all.

From pebbles to stones,
To the largest of gems,
From houses to homes,
To the very best friends.

From family to pets,
To that cozy old chair,
To umbrellas when it's wet,
To pigtails in hair.

To memories that last,
And all of those smiles,
From moments gone past,
The footprints and the miles.

Treasures are kept,
Whether remembered or framed,
Treasures are collected, boxed, and saved.

No matter the wrinkles, no matter the year,
No matter youth, whether far or near,
Treasures are sacred, whether close or far apart,
Treasures are with us, held close to the heart.

Three Little Cats

Kaitlyn Tate
Walter Hill Elementary School, Grade 1

Three little cats are my treasure because they

are special and sweet. Everyday when I come home after

school they jump up on my lap. When I'm done with my

homework I play with them, too.

Stars

Lindsey Batte
Thurman Francis Arts Academy, Grade 8

As I sit alone beneath the stars, I begin to forget the day. Every problem I had starts to wash away. I look up into the stars and start to realize how small I am. I wonder why the universe is so vast that I can see only a glimpse of its entirety. It still goes on further than the eye can see, into the black abyss. I ask God aloud, "Why is the universe so large while we are so small?"

It was like having a conversation with a dear friend. In a low, deep, calm voice, I heard from above, "For you." My heart begins to toss inside my chest, and I begin to weep. God created this universe to show how big and immense He is. It was a gift to His children to show His awesome power and glory. We should cherish this gift.

I now realize how real God is. Maybe you should take a few minutes out of your night to look at the stars. Perhaps your eyes will be opened, as mine were.

Treasures

Leah Hooper
Riverdale High School, Grade 12

I treasure human hearts. Without hearts, there would be no one living to treasure. There would be no tangible things to treasure, either. There would be no life at all, leaving nothing to treasure, not even ideas and dreams. I think a human heart is the ultimate human treasure.

My Dog

Zachary Trimm
Walter Hill Elementary School, Grade 1

My dog's name is Braden.
Braden is a white puppy.
We got him on Tuesday last year.
He is so special.
We watch him a lot because we love him.

Rejection

Kate Simpson
Thurman Francis Arts Academy, Grade 8

Rejection is such a harsh feeling;
It has confiscated me.
I went from such a happy person
To one who feels ugly.
And those who have told me boys are stupid, silly, and mean,
Have no idea how it feels to have envy turn you green.
It is not like I really care;
He just doesn't like me, that's all.
Well, if I don't care what he thinks,
Then why do I feel so small?
And I swear,
I am not a drama queen.
I just really liked him, you know,
And feeling this way has confused me...
From here, where do I go?
I know that there are many fish in the sea
And searching does take time.
But why do I feel the need
To crawl somewhere and hide?
I think we could be great,
But to him it did not seem good.
I would have treasured every moment,
Anytime I could.
But, rejection
Is such a harsh feeling;
It has confiscated me
And the hurt that I feel
Will take long until
It sets me free.

I Love...

Sara Gregory
McFadden School of Excellence, Grade 6

I love to race
Feel the wind in my face!
Without a trace.
I love to race.

I love to dance
To hop and prance!
I'll always take the chance.
I love to dance.

I love to skate
I think it's great!
I'll roll to the gate.
I love to skate.

I love to pray
Each and every day!
The Bible docs say.
I love to pray.

Treasures

Sydney Elliott
Central Middle School, Grade 8

A treasure is a gift
Kept in one's heart
That is never to be broken
Or taken apart
It may cause a tear, a laugh
Or even a smile
But it is something to remind us
Of those special times
Every once in awhile

Meaning of Treasures

Bryanna West
Wilson Elementary School, Grade 3

Treasures mean things that are important to you. One treasure is reading books you use daily. You can read really cool stories. It also means you can take journeys to places you wouldn't get to go otherwise. Some stories are read over and over again. Sometimes you're sad when the stories end. Some of the stories I've read this school year have been so wonderful!

Journeys

Julie Graham
Riverdale High School, Grade 12

The rays of the sun peeking through the blinds, the birds chirping outside the window, hearing the words, "Rise and Shine!" coming from behind the door. As I open my eyes, I see the joys of the new day. I rise, thanking God for all the journeys coming my way, from journeys that make me laugh to ones that make me cry. In the end I know I will be okay, because I have God on my side.

Hopes and Dreams

Chelsea Mayes
Central Middle School, Grade 8

As you get older your life starts to change.
People you thought you knew aren't even the same.
So now you're growing up and don't know where to go.
The world is moving so fast but you are going so slow.
You're out in the world and it's cold and mean.
Only way to get through it is your hopes and dreams.
Sometimes you'll get stuck and you won't know what to do.
But the only way out is the way through.

In the Midst of a Storm

Joy Frierson
McFadden School of Excellence, Grade 6

Hurricane Katrina
Was a horrible thing.
It did no help for anyone,
For it had no grace to bring.

People caught in Katrina
Had hope to stay alive.
It damaged many cities
And murdered many lives.

For those who heeded the warning
To move to another place,
You could tell they were frightened
Just by the looks on their faces.

1,800 people
Were killed in just a week.
And now the damaged cities
Have become antique.

I ask you to pray
For the families who have losses
And pray for the people
Who have had lost causes.

Hurricane Katrina was a terrible thing—it's true.
You're all very lucky it did not happen to you.

Life

Mike Brooks
Riverdale High School, Grade 12

I treasure the essence of life
Every day, every morning, and every night.
You never know what life may bring,
Day by day is never the same.
You can be up or you can be down.
You can smile or you can frown.
Things will not always go your way,
But tomorrow brings another day.

What Is Love?

Megan Ash
McFadden School of Excellence, Grade 6

What is love?
Is it comforting you when you're scared?
Is it thinking of holding you tight when you're not there?
Is it being happy at the sight of you?
Is it somehow knowing that everything you say is true?
Is it never having to ask "Do I love you?"
Is it always knowing that I'll always need you?
Is it knowing you are always here?
Is it knowing your tears?
Is it feeling your heart beat?
Is it knowing you're elite?
Is it just plain loving you?
I know what I think
What about you?
What is love?

My Broken Wrist

Kathryn Brittain
Smyrna Middle School, Grade 7

One time, a few years ago, my friends and I were playing on the playground at school. It was soda and snack day. I had drunk my soda and eaten my entire snack. Then I started to get thirsty. My friend, Crista, poured some Dr. Pepper in my hands and I started drinking. It was good. When she was finished with what drink was left, we started playing.

We would go to the highest step and jump on the monkey bars. My hands were sticky and the monkey bars were dry so I held on pretty good. The teachers caught us and made us stop. When they walked off, Crista and I were leaving to go to another part of the playground. The teachers weren't looking so I jumped on the monkey bars one more time. I slipped and when I tried to catch myself it didn't work.

I ended up with a fractured wrist and a bruised elbow. It was so bad I couldn't move it. I will never disobey a teacher again.

School

Ammy Cervantes
Stewartsboro Elementary School , Grade 3

> Long, wide hallways;
> Laughter;
> Pizza;
> Candy rewards;
> Happiness;
> Math and reading -
> My school.

I Like First Grade

Amelya Dorsey
Smyrna Primary School, Grade 1

I like first grade. I like school.
School is cool. First grade is fun!
We learn when we play games!
First grade is cool! I love first grade!
I have a lot of friends at school!
On Monday we go to P.E.!

My School

Emily Todd
Blackman Elementary School, Grade 2

My school is cool because you get to have a snack at 9:00. You get to play outside. You
get to meet new friends. The kids are really nice. I love my school.

School Pictures

Katelyn Caldwell
Blackman Middle School, Grade 7

> I have school pictures coming up very soon.
> I will most likely have to wait until noon.
>
> By then I will have messy hair and ketchup on my shirt.
> Oh me, why did that ketchup packet have to squirt?
>
> I think this day will be one I want to forget.
> Am I glad it's over? You bet!

I Like School

RaeLynn Dennis
Smyrna Primary School, Grade 1

I like school because we play games. We go outside. School is fun. Ms. Boe likes me! It is fun when we eat snacks. I get 100 on my work! I like to sing in music class.

My Dream

Abby Waldron
Blackman Middle School, Grade 7

Teaching is a dream I've always had.
To help kids learn makes me so glad.

I've always liked children no matter their size
and to see them learn is such a great prize.

Teach them something new every day
and helping them along their way.

There is so much more to teaching than meets the eye.
Some children are lonely, fearful, and shy.

Children need guidance, help, and care
to learn life's lessons and how to share.

To teach is a big job you can see,
but teaching would mean so much to me!

Treasures

Maggie West Harris
McFadden School of Excellence, Grade 2

I treasure my life! I just love my life!
The best thing that has happened to me is going to school and learning.
I can even remember my very first day of school.
I treasure the things I learn in school because
It will help me be a better fashion designer.
My life's dream is to be a fashion designer and to go to Paris one day.
We all want a really, really, good education. The more things I learn,
The more things I can do in my life. I'll always love my life.
I treasure my life!

"I Wonder" Song Lyrics

Olivia Zocco and Brooke Woodson
Rockvale Elementary School, Grade 8

It started in Mrs. King's second grade class
That's where I met my best friend
Third grade with Mrs. Blanton we met another girl
It started out rough, but it was all good in the end

I wonder what that day is going to be like
The day we have to say our good-byes
Everyone laughing, crying, hugging
Trying to remember all those good times

Mrs. Burnes fourth grade class was the best
She was in love with Elvis and you could tell
Our fifth grade class gave Mrs. Clark a rest
We met a girl named Kelsie and got to know her well.

I wonder what that day is going to be like
The day we have to say our good-byes
Everyone laughing, crying, hugging
Trying to remember all those good times

Middle school was scary
But a bunch of fun
Switching classes, having crushes
And books that weigh a ton

I wonder what that day is going to be like
The day we have to say our good-byes
Everyone laughing, crying, hugging
Trying to remember all those good times

Thinking back on all those memories
Wanting to make tons more
But we all know it has to end,
When we walk out of those middle school doors

From Books

Phillip Black
Siegel High School, Grade 12

From line to line, page to page,
With every word I'm becoming a sage.

When I open its cover,
This alone becomes my new lover.

It can be of fiction, science, or sport,
I'm enthralled by each and every sort.

You could call me a bookworm,
Not insulted am I by any term.

From books I've learned about history, statistics, and string theory,
But not once has one made me teary.

I've been taken from the Great Depression to 1984,
These stories only leave me wanting more.

Books are the finest things man ever wrote,
I'll leave you on that final note.

I Treasure Life

Tia Freeman
Rock Springs Middle School, Grade 7

I treasure life itself,
The sweet smell of nature when I walk out the door,
To the sight of my mom welcoming me home, I adore.

Butterflies in the morning skies,
To the moonlit night watching the lightening bugs fly.

I treasure my friends,
I will love them to the end,
Just knowing that we've been through thick and thin.

I treasure spending time with my family,
Seeing everyone enjoy each other happily.

I treasure God giving me a voice to speak,
So I thank him for making me unique.

I treasure life itself,
Yes I do,
I treasure life itself,
And that will always be true.

Poke'mon Game

John Williams
Blackman Elementary School, Grade 4

I wanted it for what seemed like forever. I finished the earlier version months ago. I cleaned my room and mowed the lawn many times. I had to earn money to buy it. Finally, I had enough money to buy it. Chuck, my older brother, took me to the store. I went in the store and had to ask a lady to open the case that had the game. She had trouble opening it, so another man came and finally was able to open it. I gave the lady my money.

When I got it, I was happy and I could barely contain myself. I jumped into the car and slid it into my game boy. I started a new game, but could not play that long. We were going to meet Mom for lunch. I was upset because my other brother Zachary would be with mom, and he really likes Poke'mon, too. I didn't want to make him mad by letting him see me play. Lunch was terrible. I had the game in the car, but I couldn't play it because I was stuck eating lunch! Finally, lunch was over.

Then, Chuck, Zachary, and I went home together. I hid myself in Mom's room. I could finally play. I was so happy! I still haven't finished the game because I don't get the chance to play much. School keeps me too busy.

My Treasures

Haily McCormick
Rock Springs Middle School, Grade 7

Where do I look? Where do I search?
Where is it that my treasure lurks?
Where do I go? Will it show?
Could my treasure be within my soul?
Or is it right there in front of me?
Is it just that I cannot see?
Will I ever know?

Do I wait and see if my treasures leave?
Or do I go and hunt them from my dreams?
Do I sit up in bed and cry with dread?
Or could it be—
My treasures are everything that makes up me!

Cub Scout Camping

Ethan Boyd
Blackman Elementary School, Grade 4

Cub Scout camping is mighty fun!
Flash light, backpack, sleeping bag and more
Fishing pole, pocket knife, going to the camp store
Walking, skipping, just don't run!

Trail mix, camping beans, burnt hot dogs
The s'mores will leave you begging for more.
Dining hall food is the best of all.
"Wednesday night ice cream is a scream!"

Canoeing, fishing, and hiking too
Sitting around the fire telling scary ghost stories
Sleeping in a tent with your snoring dad
Best of all "Mail Call!" from mother and little brother.

When you come home you feel
Like a raggedy cloth.
Muddy and tired, sore and happy
Because Cub Scout camping is mighty fun!

Chapter Two

Treasures of
Friendship

My Old Best Friend
Kacey Shepherd
Siegel High School, Grade 9

I remember when we met on the playground, underneath the hot sun.
I remember fighting over the little things.
I remember inside jokes that got us through our worst.
I remember when we danced in the pouring rain.
I remember we would laugh for hours, but only we knew what we we're laughing about.
I remember crying on each other, just because our lives didn't turn out like fairytales.
I remember being "connected at the hip."
I remember where one went the other was soon too follow.
I remember writing our lives out on paper.
I remember all the fun times we had together.
I remember letting you go, because I felt someone else was more important.
I love you, and miss you.
I hope you forgive me for all my wrongs.

I Remember…
Kayla Graham
Siegel High School, Grade 11

I remember that day on the playground,
The day we became best friends,
Even though I was new to the school,
And I thought the friendlessness would never end.
You two came over and asked me to play.
It was the moment my life changed for the better in every single way.

I remember the sleepovers and the board games,
The tree climbing and the dorky nicknames,
The long walks and even longer talks.

I remember the best moments from middle school.
You, playing pep music at your first football game,
And you, singing your heart out, on your way to fame.
The snow days we hoped and wished for,
Either to be let down or to earn a two hour delay.
We only got out of school for rain, anyway.
Spending the summer before eighth grade together, everyday,
Friends forever, we promised we'd stay.

Into eighth grade we stumbled,
Ready for high school, but not ready to grow.
We were starting to notice the last strands of our childhood starting to go.
As it came more near, the more reluctant we became.

Life was changing, nothing was staying the same.
The end of the year party we threw was a goodbye,
And also a promise to stay near,
To the friends we had made and the friends we held dear.

I remember that summer,
A summer of adventures, movie nights, and games,
Of boys, traveling, and of pain.
As the school year started, we all knew
It was going to take all we had to make it through.
It was a year of new friendships and dances,
Of new faces and of new chances,
Of lessons learned and lessons forgotten.
But never did our friendship get rotten.

I remember sophomore year,
A year of basketball games and football games and things to do,
A year of awkward moments and awkward silences, too.
Memories of you marching on the field,
We were so proud, yelling as loud as our voices would yield.
And you on the stage, once again,
We've always been there to support our best friend.

And now as the end of high school is nearing its close,
We're still the best of friends out of anyone I know.
So thanks for the laughter and the memories.
If there are any memories I will always remember, it will be these.

The Treasures of Friendship

Linda Cherry
Stewarts Creek Middle School, Grade 8

There's a miracle of friendship
That dwells within the heart.
And you don't know how it happens or where it gets its start.
But the happiness it brings always gives a special lift.
And you realize that friendship is God's most perfect gift.

My Greatest Treasure

Nick Kounlavong
Smyrna West Alternative School, Grade 11

Your love for me shines like a bright July day,
 like running across a beach with our toes in the sand
My whole being is soothed by your presence,
I love the way the moon shines in your eyes
I know that being with you there is no other pleasure.

You're always there for me no matter what I do or say,
and show our love for one another to all the land
You are as beautiful as a moonlit crescent.
I know that together there will be no lies
and compared to you there is no measure.

My love for you is like a warm day in May,
walking through the woods hand in hand.
What I say is true and not pretense
We can lie with out faces up looking at the skies,
and I'll whisper in you ear that you are my greatest treasure.

My Best Friend

Rachel Stroud
Blackman Elementary School, Grade 3

I'm writing about my best friend Devin. She was my first friend in this school. Even if we fight we always get through it. She's been my friend for three years.

Just last night, the night it was raining hard, we went to a Girl Scout meeting with all the girl scouts. We went together. Hopefully, she is my best friend for life.

Devin has been over to my house before. We always invite each other to our birthday parties. Sometimes I only invite her.

I hope we are in middle school and high school together. She is very special to me, and she is my best friend. We will always be friends.

My Best Friend

Reema Patel
Christiana Middle School, Grade 8

We have those memories,
and those great stories.

They make us laugh and make us cry,
but we go through life by and by.

She is my bodyguard and I am hers,
a fight between us hardly occurs.

She stands by me when life's bad.
She can be fierce when she's mad.

We have those jokes, inside and out
You hardly ever see a pout.

We spent together those crazy days,
and acted in those crazy ways.

Now she's moving and I will cry.
I'll be sad, but never show it, at least I'll try.

My fondness of her goes far in measure,
She will be my treasure forever.

Casie is my best friend and my treasure!

My Special Friend

Amy Gafnea
Blackman Elementary School, Grade 4

Ali, you're a special friend.
We played and laughed
And had the best of times.
We liked the same things.
We rode horses and our bikes.
But, I had to move away –
The saddest day of my life.
I think of you often and wish
Things were still the same.
You are missed, my special friend.

Best Friends
Katie Macon
Blackman Middle School, Grade 6

You are a friend
I am a friend
We are best friends

We play together
We laugh together
We learn together

If you cry, I'll be there
If you fall, I'll lend a hand
If you want to talk, I'm all ears

You are a friend
I am a friend
We are best friends

Friends Are Treasures
Sarah Cook
Thurman Francis Arts Academy, Grade 2

Good friends are treasures. My friends are very nice. I like to play with my friends at the pool and at the park. Friends are there when you are sad and need them. I like being able to tell my secrets to my best friends. If you want to have a good friend, then you need to be a good friend. That's why friends are treasures to me.

Pain Inside

Taja Cannon
Cedar Grove Elementary School, Grade 4

There is pain inside
I've got to hide
Cause my friend lied
She tried
To crush my pride
Inside

I feel like a bird in the sky
And I ask myself why
I say because she is sly
And I cry

I try to be strong
But I was wrong
Because I was gone

I try to find myself, but now I just hide
Inside
My pride
May be gone but I am still inside
And I try to keep my pain and pride
Inside

Best Friends

Taylor Hope White
David Youree Elementary School, Grade 3

Mika and I met at Tots Landing in the quiet center. We looked up and knew we were going to be friends at once! As we grew up we still were friends. Mika went camping with us every once and a while. We rode our bikes around a circle, and said "Hi" to the rangers. At night we watched a movie in the camper. Mika, my brother, my mom, my dad, and I ate breakfast. Then we had to pack up. Mika and I were sad. When we got home we played all day long.

Friends

Christine Monchecourt
Blackman Elementary School, Grade 4

Over the mountains,
Under the seas,
Across the rivers,
There's you and me.

Here we stand
Hand and hand,
Where nothing can
Break us apart.

Though if we do
Get separated,
You'll always
Be in my heart.

Friend$

Dallas Brewer
Blackman Middle School, Grade 6

My treasures are my friends…
They cheer me up when I'm sad
My treasures are my friends…
They stick with me through good times and bad
My treasures are my friends…
They are there night and day
My treasures are my friends…
They always know the right thing to say
My treasures are my friends…
They are the best
My treasures are my friends…
Together we can overcome any test

Friendship

Magen Brown
Blackman Middle School, Grade 6

Friendships are full of laughter and fun,
Sometimes they stay up till the rise of the sun.
Even though they fight,
They hate to loose each other's sight.
They talk all day and night,
and they love to have pillow fights.
Although horror movies give them a fright
They know they can sit close and hold each other right.
They like to go to each other's houses to spend the night.
That's what a good friendship is like.

Friends

Katy Appleton
Thurman Francis Arts Academy, Grade 5

Friends look out for you wherever you go.
Even through the ice, the rain, and the snow.
Sleet and hail and lightning, too;
They'll do all of that just for you.
My friends are very special to me;
Without them I have no idea where I'd be.
Take a look at us and then you will see,
What good friends we have come to be!

Friendship

Clarissa Leephone
Blackman Middle School, Grade 6

When you are sad I will dry your tears
When you are scared I will ease your fears

If you want to give up I'll help you cope
When you are lost and can't see the light,
I'll be your beacon shining so bright

This is my oath I pledge to the end.
Why you may ask?

Because you are my friend!

Friends

Khalil Kelso
Wilson Elementary School, Kindergarten

I enjoy playing with my neighbor and friend. We play cars, dump trucks, and spinning rocks with dump trucks. His name is Bryant and we have fun together.

My **Best** Friend

Emilee Peyton
Blackman Middle School, Grade 7

She's my very true best friend,
She's here until the very end.
She is there for me with everything I do.
She even makes me smile when I don't
really want to. She's my friend when I'm
in any mood, even when I am, to her, very rude.
She and I are gonna be friends forever.
I couldn't ever find anyone better.
She says the PERFECT thing at the PERFECT
time. I know she's the only reason the
sun will always shine. She is my treasure,
nothing in this world could be any better.
It doesn't matter if I win or lose, who's
there for me? Oh, Cassie Michelle Hughes.

Best Friend

Brittany Fitzgerald
Oakland High School, Grade 11

Today I met a great new friend
Who knew me right away.
It was funny how she understood
All I had to say.
She listened to my problems
She listened to my dreams.
We talked about love and life
She'd been there so it seems.
I never once felt judged by her
She never had to have her say.
She just listened very patiently,
And didn't go away.
I wanted her to understand
How much this meant to me.
I put my arms in front of me,
And when I tried to pull her near,
I realized that my new best friend
Was nothing but a
MIRROR.

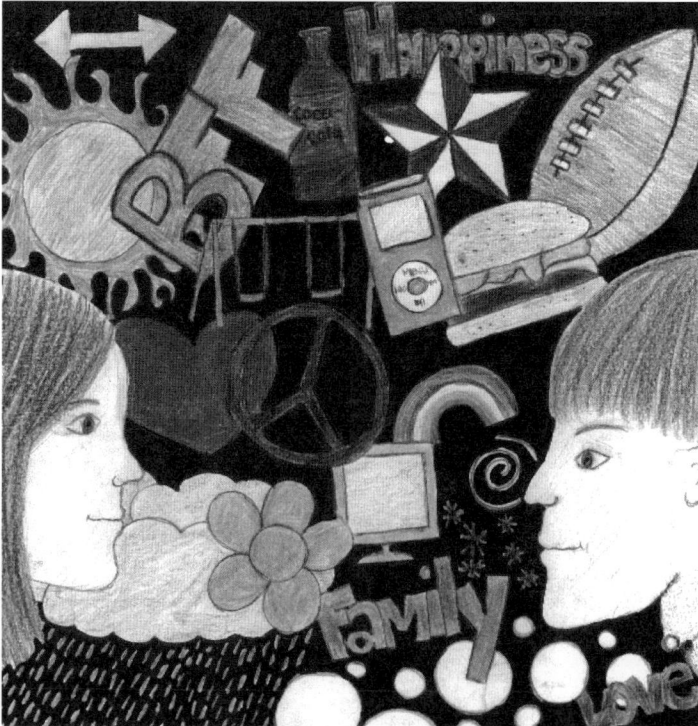

Louise King, Siegel High School, Grade 11

Always There for Me

April Freund
Thurman Francis Arts Academy, Grade 8

You tell me it will be all right when my heart is broken in two
Then you tell me, "I will always love you"
Even though we disagree
I can tell you will forever be with me
I know sometimes I do talk back
Probably then you want to give me a smack
I will always love you and
I know you will always be there for me

I love it when you're proud of me and that beaming look comes upon your face
The way your lips turn into a smile
Then actually stays there awhile
Or the way your eyes sparkle and gleam in the light
When you proudly tell me I'm bright
I know you will always be there for me

I love it when I'm scared and you hug me tight
Then repeatedly tell me it's all right
The voice you use is so calm and smooth
It is just the right sound to soothe
I know you will always be there for me

I will always love you, even when I hurt your feelings or do something wrong
Also, I'm sorry if I don't always want to bring you along
I'm getting older and won't always need you around
Though you will still tag along and stand in the background
I know you will always be there for me

I may not make the right decisions when life throws curveballs at me
But I will confidently know you will always be there for me

Dedicated to My Mom

My Best Friend

Ally Garcia
Blackman Elementary School, Grade 3

My best friend, Avery Patterson, is my treasure. She is the best thing that ever happened to me. One day I was at a basketball game and she was there. She was the one that stood by my side. While I was warming up for basketball, she wrote a story about basketball and me. It was how I could do things that a lot of other people couldn't do in basketball. I read it and at the end she cared about me a lot. So I respect that.

Avery and I will be best friends forever. I love the way we play and laugh and sing and, of course, cherish each other in the way nobody else does. We have fights, but at the end we always laugh. When she is not there, I feel really sad. I think she's really smart. She says I'm the best, but I always think she is. She is always going to be the best friend I've ever had. She is there when I fall and when somebody is being mean. She is the one that is there when I need her. She always makes me laugh. She helps me at my time of need and I love it. She is very pretty, but she says she isn't. She is very kind and helpful. Because she is my best friend, I will always like her and love her as my best friend. Avery is the person that will help me when I need it. If you know Avery Patterson, you are a very, very, very lucky person. She also plays basketball with me. She makes me smile when I'm sad. She also likes animals. When she grows up, she wants to be a photographer. She is my best friend and I love that.

Best Friends

Avery Patterson
Blackman Elementary School, Grade 3

One of my greatest treasures is Ally Garcia. She is my best friend. I met her in kindergarten. We've been best friends ever since. We have a lot of things that we both have a special passion for. We both like basketball a lot! Ally is nine, and I'm still eight. But to us, it doesn't matter about age difference. We're now in third grade. We're in the same class! We both go to Blackman Elementary School.

I'm very lucky that I have Ally as a friend! She's the person I mostly hang out with. Basketball season is coming up and she's sensational! She's the star of the court! She's not as tall as I am, but her size doesn't change her personality at all! We have a lot of laughs because she's really funny! She doesn't like dancing and cheerleading like I do, but it's okay. She has some things that she likes and I don't, but it's okay. She's really smart, too! Anyway, the whole point of me writing this is the fact that she means a lot to me.

Best Friends Forever

Brittany Lester
Oakland High School, Grade 11

I remember when we met with
pigtails and bows.

I remember playing "beauty parlor"
and painting our toes.

I remember when all there was to fight
over was who could jump the highest.

I remember sneaking in the cookie jar,
we thought we were the slyest.

I remember all the sleepovers and
late night giggles we had.

I remember catching a frog at the
pond and naming it Tad.

I remember all the tears we've shed
and the hugs we've shared.

I remember going to the doctor with
you when you were scared.

I remember starting junior high and getting
separated by classes, but we still stuck together.

I remember starting high school, side-by-side
still saying "best friends forever."

Sisters

Ashley Weber
Blackman Elementary School, Grade 4

Sisters
Caring, dependable
Sweet, loving, playing
Always there for me
Family

True Friend

Violetta Vylegzhanina
Riverdale High School, Grade 10

Whether you are sad or happy,
Whether you are tired or not,
The true friend will understand you,
And always will share your thoughts.

When you are feeling alone,
The true friend will come without fail.
He will dispel all your sadness,
And make the gladness to prevail.

When you suffer from doubts,
And do not know right way,
The true friend will come around
To throw your doubts away.

When you are ill and need cure,
The doctor would not help as well
As thought that your true friend is hear,
And putting your illness to jail.

When you can not find the solution,
And when you need the advice,
The true friend will give you the power
That not to believe to, and not to imbue
The lines of obstructions and troubles.

The true friend will never betray.
The true friend will never leave you.
The true friend will not be away.
The true friend will always forgive you...

Chapter Three

Performing Treasures

Unbelievable Peace

Kelsie Morgan
Riverdale High School, Grade 12

To some, the stage can be the scariest place in the world. . . when your hands start to shake and your stomach turns in knots. It is the most judgmental place that anybody could be, but for me it's the safest. It is the only place where I feel unbelievable peace. . . it's home for me.

Dance, Dance, Dance

Becca Baker
McFadden School of Excellence, Grade 6

Feel the rush!
Feel the thrill!
I'm working on
My favorite drill.

Change fast,
Put in a bow.
Get down and stretch,
Touch your toes.

See the audience,
At first sight.
Do the step,
Make it right!

Leap, jump, and
Turn a spin!
Do your best, get a medal
WIN!

The excitement is over,
I'm all out of breath.
All energy is gone,
I know none is left.

Mounted Treasure

Catherine E. Mote
Riverdale High School, Grade 12

The gravel crunches under the weight of a thousand pound prancing beast, as a high-pitched whinny echoes across the ground. Rider and horse stop at the gate and gaze across the rolling yellow hills of grass glazed with ice, the wind biting into their skin. The rider vaults gracefully into the saddle. Energy is high as they take off across the hills into the rising orange sun.

My Guitar

Matt Pinkston
Christiana Middle School, Grade 8

The smoke coming from the strings as I do a super fast lead
All the pitches and notes being hit
The strings as my fingers touch them
The money rolling in
I will become the best lead guitarist I can be
My music is my treasure

Dance

Simone Harris
Riverdale High School, Grade 12

Spotlight shines. . .
All eyes on me, alone.
Just me and the music.
Hear the beat. . .
Body moves along.
I know He's watching from above, pleased, smiling.
My Father in heaven.

The '06 Chorus Concert

Monique Little
Siegel Middle School, Grade 6

One warm spring evening, it was the night of the spring chorus concert and I had my first solo. I was so nervous! I could not stop shaking with fear and excitement! All of my friends and family were there to support me.

When the time came for us to go on stage my knees began to quiver. My heart was racing faster and faster. I was in complete shock; then "BAM," we were on the on the stage. While we were waiting to get on the risers I did my best to stay calm so I smiled big and began talking quietly to the people around me until the band stopped playing. Then we got onto the risers.

The first few songs went smoothly. Then, it was my turn. I began to go back into shock, but I stopped my clf just in time to get to the front of the stage. I slowly stepped up to the ice-cold microphone. There was no turning back now! My heart pounded so hard inside of me that I thought it would burst!

My voice seemed so loud in the absolute silence. There I was singing alone in front of what seemed to be 300 people and I hadn't even messed up or frozen up! I was so happy!

When my solo was over, I quickly stepped back onto the risers and took a big sigh of relief. I did it! Then I began to sing the rest of our songs. When the show was over I pushed through the crowed until I found my family. They were so proud of me; you could see it in their eyes. They told me over and over again how well I had done. My dad handed me some beautiful flowers and when we got home my mom had gotten me a marble cake with "Sing Your Heart Monique" written on it.

All in all, my solo went great! It was an amazing experience and I would love to do it again some time. I'm sure that I will not forget it!

Our Field

Shelby Leffler
Siegel High School, Grade 10

As I step back out onto the gridiron after the game
I look at the field and the stadium around me.
I can feel the power and the strength
Of the blood and sweat that was shed at practices
And the games that we have won in the past.
Claiming Our Victory!
Standing on the 50 yard line,
Looking up at the scoreboard into the lights,
Then back down at the field,
Seeing flashbacks from different plays.
I know I wouldn't have changed a thing,
Because if I did,
We probably wouldn't be the
Champions that we are today.

My Baseball Team

Logan Miller
David Youree Elementary School, Grade 3

First, when I met my baseball team it was fun. But when I met my coach he was a little nicer. At games he got ticked off a lot. After we had a game, he would give someone a game ball. I think everyone got one. At the next game, I hit the ball. It went over the second baseman's head. Then I ran the bases. Then I got stopped on third. We won. I got the game ball, finally. I hope I get a different coach each year.

Baseball

Peyton Milam
Blackman Elementary School, Grade 3

Baseball is my favorite!
And I have a lucky bat.
Slam the ball for a homerun!
Everyone cheers when we win.
But when we loose we still go out for ice cream.
All my teammates cheer.
Lucky is one teammate's name.
Look out for the ball!

Gymnastics

Beth Shirley
David Youree Elementary School, Grade 3

Gymnastics
Fun, exciting
Run, jump, bounce
You can do it
Flip, roll, fly
Fast, hard
Flipping

Baseball

Krissy Drummond
Walter Hill Elementary School, Grade 2

Baseball
And
Summer
Everyone's
Best
All time
Love in this great
Land!!

Journey to Home

Shanna Faulk
Oakland High School, Grade 10

The warm rays of the sun hit my face as I'm standing at bat.
Knuckles locked, back bent, elbows out, ready to explode.
To my left is my enemy, the ball of fate.

Hit it far or hit it deep?
A question that haunts the crowd.
Should I bunt it or go full out?
No one knows but me.

Towards the lights I try to hit, counting one by one.
The multicolored beams are blinding what I see.
The pitch is made, I dare to hit, and soaring it goes
Between the lights and screeching fans.

I don't see where else it goes, distracted as I may be.
I run to first to get the signal to go to second base.
The ball is thrown too fast for my own good, not knowing if I will get out.
Sliding in, feet first, judging by the distance, I am safe.
I get up, one foot still on base, guarding who I am.

Pop fly is hit. Toward the ground it goes.
Running as fast as lightning, passing third, and going home.
I am invincible, and nothing can touch me.

Before my eyes, I cannot believe the sight I am seeing!
The ball is thrown, nowhere to go, I cannot help but wonder.
The leather glove touches my skin, and I know that I am out.

85

Baseball

Tyler Paul
Oakland High School, Grade 11

It's the smell of hotdogs and green grass.
The joy that comes from the Little League
fields to the Major League fields.
The little kids staying up late to watch
their favorite team on T.V.
Their parents enjoy watching them
play at the sandlot.
Memories made at the field
Baseball is my treasure.

Rockvale Rattlers

Peyton Henderson
Rockvale Elementary School, Grade 3

When I was four I came to my Dad and told him that I wanted to play baseball. He is a great Dad. He said I would love to be your coach. Together we worked hard, practiced long, and helped each other. I am eight now, and we finally achieved what we worked so hard for. We took the team we built and won the Rutherford County Championship. We couldn't stop there, so we took our team further and ended up winning the title of State Championship. Our team name is the Rockvale Rattlers. This treasure of mine will never be forgotten.

Soccer

Austin Forsberg
Blackman Elementary School, Grade 4

Sport
Out of bounds
Championship
Captain of the team
Excitement because we won the game!!
Restart the game

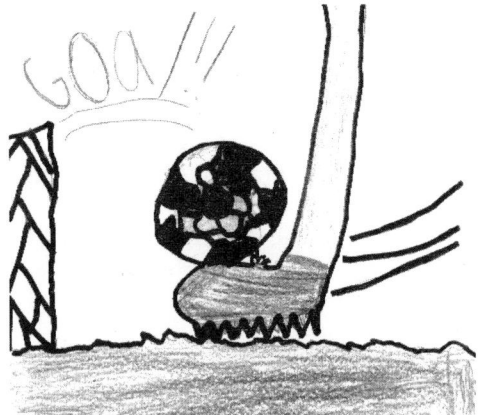

Austin Forsberg
Blackman Elementary School, Grade 4

The Baseball Hero

Adam Trigg
Wilson Elementary School, Grade 5

In our league, there are twenty-four baseball teams. Only twelve will make it to the playoffs. Only one will win it all. You have to win at least seven games to make it to the playoffs. We barely made the playoffs by winning the last game of the regular season.

We won the first two games by one point. We had it hard, but we pulled through. The game that decided if we went to the Championship was a tie all the way to the end. But, again, we pulled through two to one.

The championship game was the best game of my life. The scent of the hotdogs rushed to my nose, and the sand jumped into my eyes. The game was tied zero to zero in the bottom of the sixth inning.

I came up to the plate. "Striiiiike one!" yelled the ump. "Striiiiike two!" So there were two outs, two strikes, and it was the last inning. Here comes the pitch, and the announcer tried to distract me. It is a curveball straight down the middle. Ding!! That ball is going, going, back, back, and it's GONE! The Braves win it! The Braves win it all!

My coaches gave out medals and trophies. This would finally be the end. I felt sad because the season was over, but I also felt glad because our team won the championship game. I can't wait until next season!

My Baseball Championship

Doug Davis
McFadden School of Excellence, Grade 5

My best memory is when my baseball team won the Optimist baseball championship. We only lost one game that season, and it was against the team that we played in the championship, the Reds. Luckily, we had the best player in the league.

Noah "Freight Train" Fisher was the best player in the league, and on our team. The reason we called him Freight Train is because he hit two home-runs that year, and crushed a ball so hard it knocked a second baseman's glove clean off! The game was just about to start when it started raining. The game got postponed to June twenty-second.

In the third inning, we were down, 12-2. We scored seven runs, making it 12-9. In the fourth inning, the Reds scored seven runs, making it 16-9. We scored no runs that inning and were trailing by seven runs. We thought we were done for... Not so fast! Our pitcher, my best friend Cole, got three straight outs. We scored seven runs, making it 16-16. They scored one run and made it 17-16. In our final at-bat, we scored two runs, making it 18-17! This is the most magnificent memory of my short life.

Basketball

Emily Heyduck
Central Middle School, Grade 7

The blood, the sweat, the tears
The laughter, the cries, and cheers
Fast break, shake, and bake,
Pump fake, love, and hate
Five souls entwined as one
As if this game is to be won
Swish is like a call from heaven
As if God came down and said
Nothin' but net
Because in this league
It's not about the cash,
Or the camera flash
It's about the love of the game
And in that there is no shame
So go on get out there and score
Do it as if no one has done it before
The game decides on what you choose
So play with pride
WIN OR LOSE!

My Baseball Treasure

Rebecca Patt
Siegel Middle School, Grade 7

There is a treasure I'd like to share
It may not be a thing, but it is a memory
It happened over the summer
My treasure is the grand slam, that I made on the
16th of June
I hit it over left center's head
It went rolling to the fence
As I ran the bases, I could hear the crowd shouting
After I touched home plate my team surrounded me
That was a day I would never forget
The grand slam was awesome,
So was the first place win at the National Invitational Tournament.
In other words
We won the N. I. T.
This would have to be one of my greatest treasures.

The Baseball Game

Hope Raney
Smyrna Primary School, Grade 5

When I grow up I want to be a famous softball player. I only play "okay" for now, but I know I can do better. I've seen myself play extraordinary games, especially after a good practice with my Aunt Stephanie. My Aunt Stephanie plays for Blackman High School, and she's great. I admire her a lot. I know some day I will be one of the best, just like she is.

One of those extraordinary moments was when I was playing for the Lady Braves. We needed a first baseman, so I asked the coach if my dad could play. The coach had no other choice and put him in the game. By the third inning, it was 14 to 16, and we were the ones losing. It was my turn to bat. On the way to the plate my dad gave me some really supportive words. He reminded me of my dream and told me to reach for the stars. As I walked to the plate I started to feel better as my father's words started to sink in. I was up and ready to hit the ball. The first pitch was a ball, the next one was a strike. On the third throw, I hit it as hard as I could; I swung the bat and sent the ball flying into the outfield. I did it! I made it to second base. I knew then I would some day make my dream come true, as long I continued to practice.

Another extraordinary moment was just last year. Right before the game I went to my aunt's house to warm up. I kept hitting foul balls. It was making me madder and madder by the minute. My aunt made me stop practicing and instead took me out to eat ice cream. We laughed and enjoyed ourselves. As we headed for the game, she told me "You just needed to relax. I am sure you will now play an excellent game." I was the best that night. I didn't miss one ball.

I know some day I will be a famous ball player. In the mean time, I will continue to work hard at it and enjoy the game.

Soccer

Garrett Jakubek
Christiana Middle School, Grade 8

The ball is in the goal
Fresh cut grass
The fans are cheering
I have scored
Gator-aide in my mouth
New winners
Soccer is my treasure

My First Homerun

Nick Kristinus
Siegel Middle School, Grade 6

It was getting dark out and a storm was coming in. My team and I were in Cookeville for a baseball tournament in July of 2003. We were down 2 to 1.

It was the bottom of the seventh inning and was hot and humid. One of my teammates just got a double. Then another teammate grounded out and another. Now the entire team was down and nervous and thought we were going to lose the game. I came up to the plate and my dad told me to take a deep breath. Storm clouds were getting closer now. We heard that rain was a couple of miles away.

I now had two strikes and two outs. I did not want to strike out and have us lose the game. I was sweating and even more nervous. My dad told me to stand tall. He threw the ball. I knew it was the perfect pitch. I swung hard and felt the ball hit the bat and it felt good. I saw the ball going towards the left center field fence. Then I saw it go over the fence.

I had won the game for my team and we were going to the State championship game. We went on to the championship game but lost. I was still so happy I had hit my first homerun. We drove all the way home talking about my homerun.

It was awesome! I will never forget my first homerun. I had the ball in my hand the whole way to my house. I showed all of my friends the ball that I hit over the center field fence. All of my friends asked how far the ball went. I always had to ask my dad that question and he said that it went about 220 feet.

Now when any of my friends tell the story about my homerun I get a little smile on my face and remember how great it felt.

Thought Treasure

Paul Boykin
Riverdale High School, Grade 12

It is an eerie night, with a slight chill, not too cold to bear. A damp mist in the air, fog from the mouths of those who are breathing. Low cut grass, so fine it's almost unreal. A crowd of thousands roaring in support. A band sounding its horns. As I hear the clattering of cleats across the pavement, I know it can only mean one thing... it's game time!

Basketball Is My Sport

Ashley Stewart
Wilson Elementary School, Grade 1

My dream is to play basketball because I can be in games. I love shooting in the hoop. My cousin teaches me how to pass and shoot basketball. I meet new friends and practice skills. It makes me happy when I shoot.

Cheerleading

Emily Pack
Blackman Elementary School, Grade 4

Cheerleading
Fun, exciting
Learning, loving, trying
Cheerleading is very fun
Sport

Stereotypical Cheerleader?

Tori Craddock
Smyrna High School, Grade 11

For some time now, society has considered the stereotypical cheerleader to be blonde, stick-skinny, popular, and most of all a dim-witted girl with a reputation. Supposedly, all cheerleaders care about is their looks and the boys they are cheering for. I am here proudly declaring, "I am a cheerleader and that definitely does not describe me." I am a tall, athletic junior in high school who strives for excellence in my cheering and education. I am enrolled in many advanced honor courses, as are my cheerleader friends. I have time and time again heard the rude comments from my peers and have learned to look beyond them. Facing the stereotype is all in a day's work for me.

Many people do not know, therefore, do not appreciate the effort involved in cheerleading. Some say we are not strong, but we throw girls fifteen feet in the air and catch them with a smile. Some may say we are not smart, but we maintain our outstanding GPA's and memorize close to 100 cheers and formations. Can you jump higher and run like a track star, tumble like a gymnast, stretch like a ballerina, and take impact with NO PADS like a football player? The squad and I can.

Cheerleading is a sisterhood that continuously bonds us; we lean on each other for support. I have accomplished so much because of the trust I have in the team and our amazing coach. We put in close to thirty hours a week together. Although we can get frustrated; ultimately, it is worth the effort. You may now have more of an insight to what I do just to cheer on the team. Next time someone asks you, "Is she a cheerleader?" maybe you will say, "No, she's an athlete."

Perfect Morning

Matt Stephens
Riverdale High School, Grade 12

Perhaps the most perfect morning
Is at eight a.m.on a Saturday,
Nothing but golf and silence.

Golf Girl

Macie Meeks
Stewarts Creek Elementary School, Grade 5

I am a golf girl.
I wonder if I will be a pro.
I hear the clinking of the ball being
Hit as I walk past the driving range.
I see the ball going 100 ft.
I wish I was as good as Tiger Woods.
I am a golf girl.

I pretend I can hit 200 ft.
I feel the club in my hand when
I think about golf.
I touch the tee when I put it in the ground.
I worry that my clubs will get stolen.
I cry when someone is injured.
I am a golf girl.

I understand the ways of golf.
I try not to hit hard but smoothly.
I dream of being a professional.
I will try my hardest.
I hope people will give golf a try.
I am a golf girl.

A Diamond Day

Josh Brawley
Riverdale High School, Grade 12

One of my treasures would definitely have to be a day on the diamond. The weather's perfect, sunny, about 80 degrees. The other team's pitcher is throwing balls clocking at about 87 to 88 miles per hour. He hits 90 to 91 on occasion. The game is a pitching battle 'til the end. You being the home team and getting last at bat is a huge advantage. They take the starter out because you rocked him last inning and his pitch count is high. The reliever is average, so all you have to do is what you do best. . . and that's HIT!

I Am

Ronnie McCullough
Christiana Elementary School, Grade 5

I am a runner
I wonder if I win
I hear the starting gun
I see the finish line
I want to win
I am a runner

I pretend I win
I feel my shoe laces
I touch my bib number
I worry about losing
I cry if I lose
I am a runner

I understand if I lose
I say I'll win
I dream I'll win
I try to win
I hope I win
I am a runner

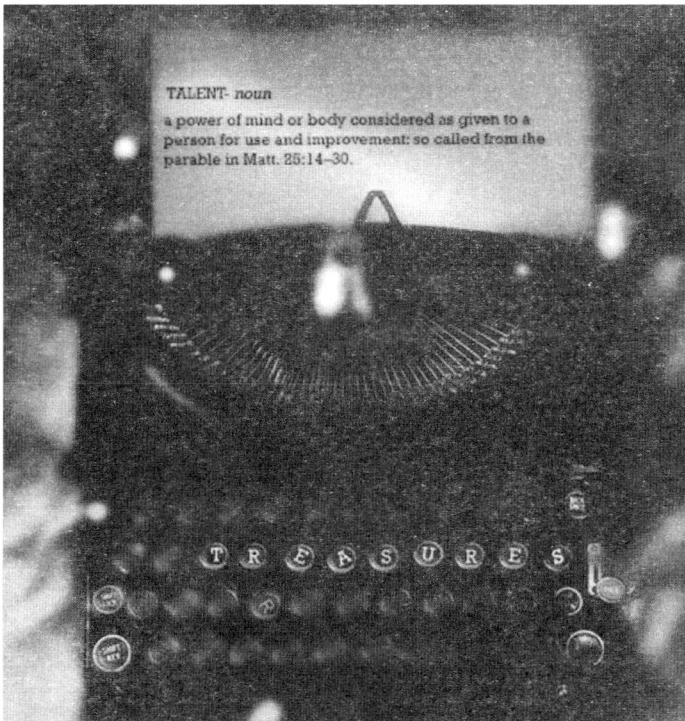

Dominique Castillo, Siegel High School, Grade 11

I Am

Gavin Burgess
Stewarts Creek Elementary School, Grade 5

I am a baseball freak.
I wonder if the Red Sox are going to win the championship.
I hear the umpire say, "Strike two."
I see Barry Bonds hit his 100th homerun.
I want to be the best player in my league.
I am a baseball freak.
I pretend that I am Barry Bonds.
I feel the ball hit the bat.
I touch the ball when I pitch.
I worry if someone gets hurt.
I cry when I get hit in the stomach by a 30 mile an hour ball.
I am a baseball freak.
I understand if we lose.
I say, "Good game," to the other teams.
I dream about being Barry Bonds.
I try again if I mess up.
I hope I will play my whole life.
I am a baseball freak.

Band Geeks Rule

Addy Rivenbark
Blackman Middle School, Grade 6

Band geeks rule!
They rule every school!

We practice everyday
We are proud to say
We are here to stay

We are heard behind the door
We definitely rock the floor

Band geeks rule!
They rule every school!

Band Competition Days

Gracie Bryson
Siegel High School, Grade 11

We arrive at the crack of dawn.
Practice…
Drilling, cleaning, public humiliation, gush and go,
"Do it again." "What were those checkpoints?" "Guard, what are you doing?"
left, right, left
BAND TEN-HUT…
We stop in our tracks listening with attentive ears
…BAND DISMISSED.

We hastily jump in our uniforms and slick back our hair and eat.
We're having pizza with a side of hairspray and glitter.
"Don't forget your shoes and gloves."

The band all piles in four yellow busses while preparing ourselves for an intense night.
The guard puts on pounds of makeup to be seen a mile away.
It would be a chore to create the perfect face on the bumpy ride had our steady hands
not done it a million times before.
The sabre line and drum line re-tape metal and wood.
Off with the old and on with the new.
In an instant the bus is silent; fifteen minutes until our arrival.
We run through the show in our heads…
Up on count 10, caddy at 3, tempo change to 140, eighth notes, rests.

We scuttle out of the crowded bus.
More practice…
"Remember, it's a caddy, not a side drop." "Don't rush!" "Adjust to the wind."
5,6,7,8

The guard gets in a huge circle and links hands.
All forty-two of us girls and our instructor huddle close.
Words of encouragement and wisdom are exchanged…
"I'm so proud of you girls." "Make this performance better than the last." "This is what
we practiced for." "Smile."
We close sending a prayer to heaven.
Guard ten-hut.

SHINE!

We gather our equipment and strip off our warm jackets to begin the voiceless trek to
the stadium.
We walk in two straight lines with nerves gone haywire.
There is excitement and nervousness, and we look confident.
When we reach the gate the directors let out one last piece of advice.
"Do you see the sign? Checkpoint City."

We go to the side lines to set up our flags and sabres.
We have our backs to the judges, facing the band entering from back field.
With our first step on the field we project to the judge's box.
We hear the question…
"Drum major, is your band ready?"
Then we hear the parent fan club with a resounding
"They're always ready!"
Siegel Band, you may take the field in competition.
"DUP, DUP, DUP, DUP"
"JUICE!"
And we begin.

Gifted

Sabrina Bradley
Rockvale Elementary School, Grade 6

It's fun having a big brain
But it can grow to be a pain
Everybody expects more of you
Even when you're just two
They always compare grades
It's always a race
When the finish first they rub it in your face
If you have homework and they don't
You're the prey for the bullies tomorrow
So next time you pick on a geek
Think about what they will go through next week

Perfect Moment

David Spurlock
Riverdale High School, Grade 12

The perfect moment. . .
The smell of cut grass. . .
Walking onto the field
For your first game.

Chapter Four

Holiday Treasures

The Time I Treasure Most
Kristia Bravo
Christiana Middle School, Grade 8

"Wake up! Wake up!", my sister screams, "Merry Christmas Kristia!" We dash down the stairs to see an empty glass, cookies ¾ eaten, and a living room filled with presents from that good ol' St. Nick...

All people have a special something that they treasure, whether it's a loved one, a memory, their hopes and dreams...That feeling I get at Christmas is what I treasure most.

Various aromas of Christmas sweetness waft from Grandma's oven: gingerbread, sugar cookies, and brownies, create crowds of family in the kitchen. Meanwhile, she hollers for them to stop getting underfoot. Even still, they cannot resist the tempting smells of her pumpkin pie, along with her other famous addictive sweets.

Visiting with family on Christmas Eve gives a comforting feeling. I love giving thoughtful presents to loved ones, and in turn, receiving the gift of expressions of joy and appreciation on faces. Of course, *opening* presents is not bad either, or getting a visit from that jolly, fat man, also known a SANTA!

Viewing sparkling, iridescent lights, recalls times of earlier childhood. Our family tradition is to make an excursion to the Opryland Hotel; therefore, I have to tolerate the taking of a billion and one pictures. Thank you *dear* Dad. Nevertheless, the dazzling lights help me to bear it.

SNOW! That white, fluffy, cotton-looking precipitation that permits making snow angels, snowmen, or just having a snowball fight. It allows fun for all ages; I am its number one fan. Just imagine, after having a long play date with snow, then coming inside to a cup of steaming hot cocoa and a nice book to curl up with.

As I have described, the smells, gathering with family, Christmas lights, and snow add up to just the greatest sensation one could ever feel. That being said, Christmas is the time of year I treasure most. Are you dreaming of a white Christmas?

A Fall Day
Kara Marie Martin
Blackman Middle School, Grade 6

The pumpkin and spice aroma in the air,
The sound of the leaves crunching under my feet,
The clear blue sky,
A cool light breeze,
All are fall's treasures.
A day off of school to enjoy fall's beauty...
The BEST treasure of all!

Fall
Jason Lorigan
Central Middle School, Grade 7

I hear the leaves crackle under my feet.
The days are growing colder.
Squirrels gathering nuts, winter's chill to beat.
Colors growing bolder.
Good things baking for me to eat,
And I am getting older.
There's no time quite as sweet.
Leaves in awe their beholder.

Thanksgiving Time Is a Special Time
Harleigh McNeely
Blackman Elementary School, Grade 2

Thanksgiving is a special time of the year. Families getting together and spending time with each other. There's lots of food to eat like turkey, dressing, green bean casserole and salad. For dessert there is lemon lush, cake, chocolate pie and ice cream.
So here's to all of the families...have an excellent Thanksgiving!

Thanksgiving Thoughts

Jane Waddington
Blackman Elementary School, Grade 5

Thank you for being polite
Having a turkey for dinner
Aunts and uncles come to visit
Need to prepare for dinner
Kisses for lots of love
Say nice things
Giving thanks for Thanksgiving
Interesting facts to learn about Thanksgiving
Visit other family
I need to eat your turkey
Neat and tidy table
Generous and forgiving

Thanksgiving

Joey Hughes
Blackman Elementary School, Grade 3

Every Thanksgiving I go to my aunt and uncle's house. My cousins and I play around until it is time to eat. Then, we eat a delicious meal. We eat turkey and dressing. We also eat ham. Then, we play a football game. It's called the Turkey Bowl. After the game, we choose the MVP! After that, we go to back to my aunt's and uncle's house. Sometimes my cousins come home with me. I feel tired, but happy on Thanksgiving. I love being with my family on Thanksgiving.

Thanksgiving Fun Day

Lauren Stafford
Blackman Elementary School, Grade 2

This is what I am going to do on Thanksgiving. I am going to my Nana and Papa's house. I'm going to eat lunch there and play. I bet my cousins are going to be there. I think there is going to be turkey-I love turkey. I am going to give my family Thanksgiving presents. I am going to give my mom a card. I am going to give my dad a picture of a turkey. That is my story.

Thanksgiving Day

Shane Schneider
Lascassas Elementary School, Grade 5

Every Thanksgiving Day
In my heart, there is a parade.
Spending time with my family
Even with good Aunt Pammy.
It is a good tradition
I love this celebration.
It's a good kind of love we share
It's a love that is very rare.

What I Did on Thanksgiving

Kendall Clark
Blackman Elementary School, Grade 2

I was going to my Grandma's house. We had a big turkey. It was fat and yummy. We had other food too. I ate my food. Then I played with my big brother. First we played tag. Next we played hide and go seek. Then we stopped playing. We went in and got a drink and Mom said to rest a minute. So we did and went home.

Christmas

Lee Russell
Blackman Elementary School, Grade 5

Christ
Hope for Santa Claus
Remember special times
I bake cookies and brownies
Sing songs about Christmas
Thankful
Many gifts
All the snow you can play with
Special day

Christmas

Lon Latimer
Lascassas Elementary School, Grade 1

I remember when I had the best Christmas ever! I got a fork lift and my cousins came to visit. I got some tinker toys. It snowed about one inch. We played in the snow!

My Best Christmas

Jordan Newman
Blackman Elementary School, Grade 4

The best Christmas ever was the year 2006. My two front teeth were missing and it was funny. There was a song called "All I Want for Christmas Is My Two Front Teeth." When I tried to sing it, it sounded weird. When I went to see Santa Claus, he couldn't understand what I wanted. I asked him for a T.V. and it came out as "V.V." On Christmas morning, I was surprised because under the tree was a stereo.

Christmas

Kyle Stroud
Blackman Elementary School, Grade 5

Carols all around
Houses lighting up
Reindeer in the sky
In the bag lots of toys
Snow on the ground
Toys under the tree
Many many goods around
And
Saint Nicholas coming down

Our Christmas Tradition

Jamia Bazemore
Blackman Elementary School, Grade 3

Every year on Christmas my family comes to my house. While we are waiting for everybody to get there, we play Monopoly. After everybody arrives, we have our Christmas feast, and eat lots of stuffing! Other things we eat are green beans, turkey, apple pie and mashed potatoes. It is always so much fun!

After dinner, we go outside and play tag. Then, we get ready to go to bed. We always sleep in the bonus room. When we are ready for bed, we get to open one present. Before we go to sleep, we watch "The Christmas Story." I'm really happy to have my family over every Christmas.

Christmas Day

Danny Rome
Blackman Elementary School, Grade 3

Christmas day is when all my family comes to my house. We have a lot of fun! We have snowball fights. We make snowmen on my dad's truck, and once we went ice-skating. Sometimes we just sit by the fire and play games and drink hot chocolate. The best thing is that I am with my family.

Christmas Dinner

Joanna Nyland
Smyrna High School, Grade 10

Imagine, a bone chilling winter's day in the middle of Christmas break. What is better than that walking around the village green in the grey shadows of dusk, the crooked, spooky spires starring down at you from the rooftops of a local church, opening the door to a house and stepping inside to a warm cozy living room? All at once, the smell of homemade cooking, tinged with a hint of smoke from an open fire hits you. I know as soon as I walk in, that my aunt has made my favorite meal. On a cold winter's evening, with frost creeping up the windows, there is nothing better to have than to have a roast dinner. A roast dinner is made up of succulent roast beef, cooked to perfection, creamy mashed potatoes that melt in your mouth, roasted potatoes, crisp garden peas, warm juicy carrots and warm, rich gravy. All this is accompanied by Yorkshire Pudding, a bread of sorts, buttery on the inside, with a golden crisp coating on the outside. It is as light and fluffy as a cloud in the sky. As I eat, I hear the babbling stream of conversation from all around me as my cousins dig into their food, piled high on their plates. The excited conversation, the occasional shout of argument from my siblings, and the peals of giggles that surround me make this meal special. A roast dinner takes all day to make, with as much effort and love put into it by those who work hard to make it such a wonderful meal. I know that this food will be gone as soon, if not before, it is put on the table.

Tiger Butter
Shannon Jones
Smyrna High School, Grade 10

Blanketed with peanut butter and white chocolate fur and lined with milk chocolate stripes, it is no wonder our family's Christmas favorite is intriguingly named "tiger butter." It is a warm, soothing scent that fills the kitchen at the holidays just before all the relatives start packing in. Tiger butter is a family tradition that, in my mind, is associated with the warmth of home and family. Its rich flavor and sweet smell hold the same sentimental holiday importance as the tree or the tinkle of bells and low hum of Christmas carols. Perhaps it is so loved by our family because of the fun that goes into making it. Every year, my brother, my mother, and I wrangle all the ingredients together. The kitchen becomes full and magnificently chaotic. The clatter of spoons, mixers, and pots fills the already crowded air of the small room. There is always the occasional swatting away of the hands of my brother and me, as we reach to lick the candy covered spoons. It is always followed by the lighthearted laugh of my mother. The smells, laughs, and even the discord of noise puts all those involved in a more festive mood. However, the best part about tiger butter is the satisfying finished product, a warm square of peanut butter and white chocolate, with milk chocolate tiger stripes swirled in, and a pecan as its heart in the center.

Krystals and Taco Soup
Jack Jones
Lascassas Elementary School, Grade 4

On Christmas Eve, my friends come over to celebrate with my family. My mom makes taco soup and my friends bring the Krystals. We play in my room and my sister's room. We watch a Santa Claus tracker on the computer. We dance, watch television, swap presents, and talk about what we want for Christmas. We draw pictures, play board games, and make cards for Santa Claus. I always put out cookies and milk. We shake our presents to guess what is in them. Finally, my sister and I go to bed. I listen for footsteps on our roof and then fall asleep. When I wake up in the morning, I open my presents from my parents and Santa. Oh what a special time!

Holiday Treasures
Hannah Mae McCravy
Lascassas Elementary School, Grade 5

On Christmas Day
People come to my house
To eat and play,
Sing Christmas songs
Open some presents
Drink egg nog!

On Halloween
I dress up
And go trick-or-treating
I eat candy
Like smarties and
Sandy candy.
There are ghosts
That are scary
And there's witches
That are hairy!

On Thanksgiving
I eat and eat all kinds of treats
Turkey, pumpkin pie, cranberries, and even rye.
The sun is shining
The skies are blue.
No one is whining...
They're all too cute!

On New Year's Eve
People love to party
They never leave!
With their party hats and balloons
People just party like wild coons!
They eat and drink
They watch fireworks
It's such a TREAT!

I love my birthday
And I love that word
It is on the day of July 23rd.
My family sings "Happy Birthday"
They cut the cake.
I blow out the candles
It's fun for goodness sake!

Special Times Thanksgiving Poem

Savannah Welch
McFadden School of Excellence, Grade 5

Thanksgiving time is almost here
It's when all my favorite foods appear

Turkey, ham, and wonderful deserts
Please don't spill gravy on your shirt

All of my family gets to come over
In the center of the table I put green clovers

It's the time where we come together
And nobody cares about the weather

Thanksgiving time is almost here
It's when all my favorite foods appear

We're drawn by the smell of sweet potato crunch
My grandma's specialty, but we don't get some 'till after lunch

The stuffing's always so delicious
It's so good it seems suspicious

Pecan pie is so sweet
Everyone wants some to eat

Thanksgiving time is almost here
It's when all my favorite foods appear
The Caesar salad is made just for me
It tastes so sweet I yell, "Yippee!"

I thank the Lord every day
When I bow my head and pray

Thanksgiving time is almost here
It's when all my favorite foods appear.

Christmas

Noah Buckley
Blackman Elementary School, Grade 4

Christmas, oh, Christmas
What joy it is!
The smells, the sights, and sounds.
When people come together
Time for family and friends.
What joy it is!
We wrap our gifts
We sing and dance to the music.
Santa is soon to come,
Giving presents to everyone.
In the morning we open our presents,
So happy, so much fun.

Cookie Cutter Memories

Chelsea Lamb
Eagleville School, Grade 12

Going to my Mammy's is always fun, especially near Christmas when there's baking to be done.

We can hardly wait as we drive up the road; the hearts in our chest are about to explode.

We look through the glass as we approach the door; our grandmother is busy sweeping the floor.

She has worked all afternoon preparing the dough; the grandchildren all rush in and she begins to glow.

With loving instruction and a watchful eye, we begin our process with a giggle and a sigh.

The old tin cookie cutters are a favorite of mine, we always pick out our favorite design.

Snowmen, angels, stockings, and wreaths just to name a few; Chad's the most creative of the whole crew.

Filling my senses as they bake, a time-honored tradition for goodness sake!

The icing and sprinkles are ready to spread, but everyone agrees their favorite color is red.

Once again we've made them too pretty to eat, so we sit back and admire our delectable treats.

We clean up our mess and say our good-byes. Mammy stands at the door and begins to cry.

Wonderful Christmas Memories

Jasmine Wakefield
Barfield Elementary School, Grade 3

C: I make **cookies** with my mom on Christmas Eve. We deliver them to my neighbors and my best friend. After that, we give the rest to our church. Everybody thinks they are very good. I can't wait until we get to make more!

H: My favorite **holiday** is Christmas. My mom loves it too. My favorite part about Christmas is when I get presents. My second favorite part is getting to see my family. I am looking so forward to seeing everyone.

R: **Reindeer** is my favorite animal. My mom and I were driving around and we saw a reindeer one Christmas. I had never seen one before. It was so pretty. It had a lot of fur, and pretty antlers.

I: When it's cold outside, I see **icicles** on my house. I think the icicles are pretty and clear. The icicles hang about five inches from the roof. I love cold weather.

S: I love to get presents from **Santa**. I leave out cookies and milk for Santa. In the morning it is all gone.

T: On Christmas Eve, my mom and I decorate our Christmas **tree**. My mom does the top where I can't reach. I tell her thank you. After we get all the decorations on the tree, she lets me put the angel on the top. It looks beautiful when it is all done. Decorating the tree is a very special memory.

M: **Merry** means happy. I am merry that my mom finally got her office cleaned out. It looks a lot better. I love when Santa says "Merry Christmas."

A: **Angels** are pretty on the top of a tree. My mom and I always put an angel on our tree. The angel we have lights up. I love angels watching over us.

S: When it **snows**, I call my friends and they come over to play. First, we have snow ball fights. Then, we build a snowman. We leave the snowman outside until it melts. When we are finished playing outside, we go in for some hot chocolate. I always put marshmallows in mine. I love snow.

Chapter Five

Family Treasures

Priceless

Zachary Shugan
Blackman Elementary School, Grade 5

Video game . . . $50.00

Football . . . $20.00

Great family . . . priceless

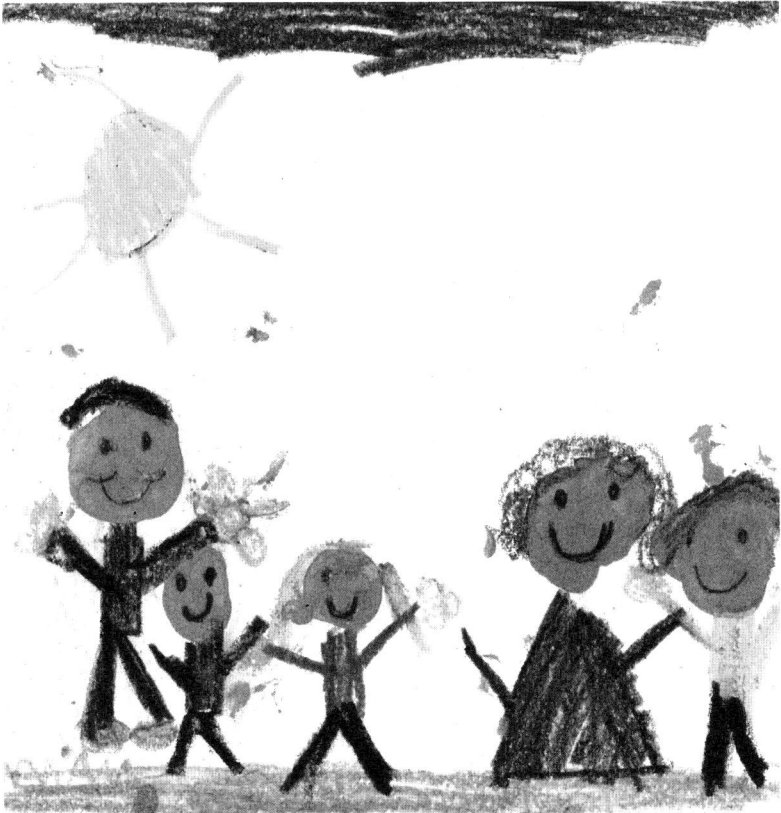

Gracie Milam, Blackman Elementary School, Kindergarten

Treasures

Mary Layne Harrell
Siegel High School, Grade 12

It was Christmas Eve, and Lissa Melbourne was standing by the kitchen counter, gazing around the dimly lit room. It was routinely decorated for Christmas, and she examined how her mother's intricate figurines were reflected in the light of the candles placed strategically throughout the room. She drew in her breath, and a wave of cinnamon, and apple, and vanilla, wafted through her nostrils. She walked across the room to the kitchen table, and pulled out a chair to sit down. She grasped a glass figurine of a carefully crafted polar bear in her hand, and studied it intently. How had her mother made the features of the polar bear so lifelike? She could practically imagine the image coming to life in her hand. She wished desperately it would, if only so that something living and breathing would be there to comfort her, something her own mother had made. Tears welled up in her eyes as she clutched the polar bear tightly. Looking around the room, she saw pieces of her mother in every direction. A glass-blown blue and black penguin perched by the phone, its expression eerie in the light of the candle directly beside it. A pale blue enamel dolphin shone from its position near the microwave. A dozen other figurines caught her eye, and Lissa felt a glow of hope grow inside her. The figurines were so real, so vibrant, how could she not feel hope for her mother's condition in each one of them? Each and every figurine had become a treasure to her, something she desperately needed in the uncertainty that plagued her on a daily basis. She pushed in her kitchen chair and slid down beneath the counter to sit on the floor, her bare feet touching the cold kitchen tile. She wondered about her mother, in that moment. It was a rare moment in which she was alone to reflect on her feelings. Someone was always there with her, whether it was her father, or her sister, or her grandmother. Lissa was thankful for their presence, but tonight, somehow the silence felt cathartic. She was alone with little pieces of her mother, figurines that had been borne of her mother's artistic talent and skill. She slowly drew up from her position on the floor and walked around slowly, cradling various figurines in her arms. She returned to her spot on the floor and placed them around her in an uneven circle. She didn't know how long she had been sitting there, reflecting on her mother, when the door burst open and her grandmother walked inside. She looked down at Lissa with wonder. She set down her packages on the counter and went to sit beside her granddaughter. "Lissa, honey," she whispered. "I miss her too." Lissa fell into her grandmother's arms, as silent tears slid down her cheeks. "She's truly gifted," her grandmother continued, stroking Lissa's shiny dark hair. "All of her work is beautiful. I never dreamed that my child would be an artist. Neither your grandfather nor I ever had a bit of artistic talent. Then your mother was born. I could tell from the first time she picked up a paintbrush that she would be an artist. And her figurines are truly some of the most beautiful pieces I have ever seen." Lissa nodded. "They are my treasures," she said in a stifled voice. "They're the only parts of her that remain at this point." Her grandmother's dark eyes bored into Lissa's. "Lissa...all hope is not gone for your mother. The doctors are anticipating a good recovery, if only..." Lissa finished for her. "If only she comes out of her coma." Lissa grasped her grandmother's hand as she answered, "She very well might, Lissa. We cannot give up hope." Lissa looked down at the figurines crowding her. "These are my hope," she said. "They somehow make me feel as though she can't be entirely gone, because so much of her remains here. I can see her personality, her touch, in all of them." Lissa's grandmother nodded silently. She too examined the figurines in the flickering light, and a bond of understanding formed between them. After several long moments, Lissa's grandmother turned to her. "We can't spend the entire night pondering about your mother, Lissa. Your sister and father will be home soon, and we still have our tradition to carry out!" Her words produced a weak smile from Lissa. "Come on, Lissa, the ingredients await," she cajoled her granddaughter. "And I know that nobody can make gingerbread as mean as ours!" Lissa had to smile widely at that. Their gingerbread was notorious for being the family's least favorite item, but the two of them snacked on it constantly during the Christmas festivities. "Okay," she said, wiping away her tears and getting to her feet. "Let's get started!" Her grandmother helped her place the figurines back in their appropriate places, and then the two of them ambled toward the refrigerator, ready to begin a whole new batch of Christmas cookies.

My Brother, My Treasure
Hayley Dawson
Christiana Middle School, Grade 7

My brother, Ian, is very important to me. He used to live here in Tennessee and work with my mom at Nissan, but he quit his job to serve his country. He works in the army as an unmanned aerial vehicle pilot. In other words, he flies huge, remote control airplanes.

Ian is stationed in Georgia where he lives with his wife and adopted daughter, and on Thanksgiving Day he will have a new daughter. Soon after the baby is born, he will have to ship out to Iraq, but hopefully not until after Christmas. He won't get to see his new baby or his family for at least a year once he ships out.

When he does go to Iraq, I will miss him a lot and pray that he doesn't get hurt. I'm very proud of my brother; I am glad he joined the army to fight for us, and I love him very much. He is my treasure and my country's treasure.

Making Cookies
Kevin Bean
Roy Waldron School, Grade 2

"Wow! Let's go make cookies," said my mom. My mom is a treasure to me because she always makes cookies with me. She also is a treasure because she gets me to school on time. She always says, "I love you." She gives me kisses and hugs all the time. I tell her I love her, too. She gives me a bandage when I scrape my leg or arm. She helps me when I fall down. She gets me to bed on time. I will always love my mom forever!

My Days as a Child

Leatha Kee
Smyrna Middle School, Grade 7

When I was born, my parents had split up. So I lived with my mom for about three years. But one day, out of the blue, I said I want my daddy. So she called my dad and told him to come pick me up. Well, he came and took me and I never saw her again.

Years have passed and my dad married Sarah. She is now my step-mom. We did run into my mom one day at the store. Well, she and my dad started fighting over who I would live with. So they ended up having to go to court and solve everything. So from this point on, I visit my mom on weekends and I live with my dad.

Even today, my mom gets mad at me for not being there with her. I love my mom and dad to death and every holiday they fight over who am I going to stay with. I just run to my room and start crying because it upsets me and I'm afraid that something might happen. But on holidays, my mom yells at me on the phone on who am I to stay with. Sometimes I just wish that they will just be together and not be mad at each other and fight.

I just thank the Lord that they are still here and that nothing will happen.

My Loved Ones!

T.J. Harrison
Smyrna Primary School, Grade 3

I'm going to tell you about my family. My mom is a hard-working mom and she cares about everything and everyone in the work except strangers. My dad is very nice, strict, and playful. My little brother, Alex, is a pain, but I don't know what I'd do without him. Now my baby brother Ryan is another story, because all he ever does is cry, eat, laugh, and go to the bathroom. My cousins are really nice and sweet to all their friends. Now, when it comes to sharing, they don't quite understand a whole lot. My older cousins are funny, silly, and understanding. My grandparents are a lot of fun. They'll play with you, eat with you, and everything else that grandparents do. If you meet my family you'll have a blast! Most important, I love my family and I always will. This story comes from my heart.

My Brother Is an Angel

Joshua Parker
Cedar Grove Elementary School, Grade 1

I had a brother named Chris. He was older than me. He was in high school. He died in a car wreck and he is an angel now. I don't remember a lot about him but my mom and dad told me I was his best friend. I loved him very much and he taught me a lot. It was nice to have a big brother. He played video games with me. When he died I was sad. When I grow up I want to be an astronaut because that was his dream and he did not get to do it. My mom tells me the stars are angels peeking down from heaven to check on us. I know Chris watches over me.

Scary Days

Corey Smith
Smyrna Middle School, Grade 7

One time in my life when my daddy and my momma were living together they used to always argue every day, night and morning. They used to wake me up at nighttime or in the early morning because they were so loud.

One morning, my momma wouldn't let my daddy out of the house and she cut my daddy in the arm. Then my daddy took the knife out of her hand and went outside and flattened her tires and moved to a hotel. That's when our family broke up.

About a year later, I moved in with my daddy. About a week later, he got locked up. Then I went back with my mommas. She didn't have a house, so I moved around in my momma's car. Then I moved in with my granny for about two months.

Later, my daddy got out and I moved back with him in 2005. I am still with my dad, and, although it's not great, it is good.

My Grandmother

Kaylee Dixon
Cedar Grove Elementary School, Grade 3

My grandmother is so special to me. She tells me stories. She's so nice to me. I call her and she says "Hi, how was your day?" When I come over she lets me watch TV. She gave me a chair that is my favorite chair. She gave me a plate and I love it and it will never fall. She is my dad's mom. We come over for Thanksgiving and Christmas. I love her!!!

The Things I Love

Caleb Lay
Christiana Elementary School, Grade 3

I love my grandfather. He was in World War II. He is so awesome and special and he even flew a bomber in the war! My grandfather was the co-pilot. This bomber was called the B-17. The most capacity it could hold was seven people. He still lives in Knoxville, Tennessee. He is very cool.

My mom and dad are also very cool. They make me mind, and they try to make me be kind to others. I try to do it, but a lot of times I don't. Sometimes they have to ground me when I don't listen to them. I love them.

The Presence of Divorce

Brandon Musgrove
Smyrna Middle School, Grade 7

A long time ago, I was probably three or four years old, my mom and dad were getting a divorce. We moved a couple of miles away. We lived in Omaha, Nebraska.

On my fifth birthday, I had a birthday party. I was so happy, because my dad was coming and I could not wait to see him. The party was from 12 p.m. to 3:30 p.m. The party had just started and I was having fun. Later, around 1 p.m., I said, "Mom, is my daddy coming?" My mom didn't answer me. So I thought yes, he's my dad he would come to my birthday party.

Three o'clock came and my dad was not there. Everyone began to leave around 3:30. The presents were being packed up and the clean up was underway. Me? I was crying. I hadn't seen my dad.

When I became nine years old, I saw my dad twice a year. We had moved again and I lived in Tennessee. Every time I visited him, it was only four days long. Then, my dad told my mom that he didn't have the money to pay half the plane ticket to Nebraska. My mom said that she wasn't paying for it by herself. So I didn't get to see him.

Now, I am 13-years old and I was supposed to go to my dad's on November 8, 2007. But he, again, did not have the money so I get to go at a later date. And he said, "He didn't know about Christmas."

So now, I wonder when I will get to see my dad. Christmas? Why? When? Why didn't he come to any of my football games like he said he would? Why? When will I get to see him again?

Grandma Is My Treasure

Hayley Royal
Christiana Middle School, Grade 8

I love the aroma of her food
Her mac and cheese is oh so good
And even though she's been through a lot
Sorry for herself she is not.

She likes the mountains and the beach
Where anything is within your reach
She's always busy never sitting
And doesn't really care for knitting.

She watches "Mama's Family" on t.v.
Sometimes she acts just the slightest bit crazy
Whenever you need her she's always there
It's nice to know she really does care.

She and I will never part
I'll love her forever with all my heart
I love to hear her stories told
Treasured memories always unfold.

She's always there in my time of need
And teaches me to always succeed
She's the very best grandma around
No other like her can be found.

My Mom

Jessy Pellegrino
Cedar Grove Elementary School, Grade 5

I love my mom with all of my heart.
She has been there from the start.
She helps me through the good and the bad.
I know she loves me, even when I make her mad.
She is my mom, I'm happy to say.
I hope to grow up and be like her some day.

My Family
Miller Armstrong
Blackman Elementary School, Grade 4

I treasure my family because it is fun camping with them. I like being in a bunk bed with my brother. I like wrestling with my brothers. I really like it when we have parties and a bon fire. It's fun sometimes when we just watch movies and chill out or when we go hiking. Overall I just like being with my family.

Loved Ones
Kacey James
Blackman Elementary School, Grade 2

I love my mom and dad so much. My mom likes to play with me. My dad goes to football games with me. I also love my grandparents. My grandma is nice. My grandpa picks me up from school. I really love my family. They mean the world to me.

My Family
Madeleine Lee
Blackman Elementary School, Grade 3

Magnificent
Young at heart

Loving
Outstanding
Vivid
I adore my family
Never gives up
God is #1

Faithful loving family
Amazing
Marvelous Memories
Inspire me
Loving Laughter
You would love them.

A Special Brother

Tiffany Quigley
Blackman Elementary School, Grade 2

I love my brother Tanner and he loves me. He gives me toys for Christmas. Sometimes he protects me and he plays with me. He also helps me with my homework. Sometimes I surprise him with presents because he is such a special brother. He is absolutely the best brother in the world.

Spivey Family Reunion

Josie Spivey
Blackman Elementary School, Grade 3

On the first weekend in November, my family goes to west Tennessee for a family reunion. We get to play with our cousins and stay in a cabin. We also roast marshmallows. Sometimes, we get to ride horses. That is one of my favorite parts! I see a lot of my relatives, and eat yummy food all weekend. Sometimes, we try to catch fish at the pond. At the end of the day we have to go to bed, but we get up the next day and go to the lodge and eat more good food! We eat the best rolls ever, really yummy spaghetti, and drooling vanilla ice cream. After we eat, we go play on the playground. I feel loved because I get to see my family.

My Treasure

Liam Elam
Blackman Elementary School, Grade 1

My treasure is my family. I have in my family mom, dad, sysr and me. I love thim.

My Grandma

Emily Yeatts
Blackman Elementary School, Grade 4

My Grandma is very special to me. When I was little she would watch me every Friday. Sometimes she would take me to Target. One time she got me a pair of Barbie Doll pajamas and some matching ones for my Barbie Doll.

My Grandma made me something really special that I still hve today. It's a blanket! My Mom said that when the edges broke my Grandma would sew it back together for me. It's so special that if it broke into a million pieces I would save all the pieces! Now it's all holey and fragile. I sleep with it every night.

Whenever I was three she died. I really miss her!

The Treasures of My Life

Christopher Whisenant
Cedar Grove Elementary School, Grade 4

I have a lot of treasures in my life. Three of my most important treasures are people. I will never forget them. I will always hold them close to my heart. They are my treasures of my life.

I love my baby sister. I will look at her and she will give me a funny look, so I give her one back. She makes me laugh and smile. She is my baby sister. I love my baby sister.

My mom is the best. She buys me most of the stuff I want or need. She makes the best boiled eggs. She loves me very much and she tries to be the best mom possible. I love my mom.

My dad is so enthusiastic about the work I do. He helps me when I am stuck. He sure makes some good steak. He rides my bike with me. He tries to be the best dad possible. I love my dad.

Treasures are the best memories you can have. They can be people or things. I am so lucky to have three special people to treasure in my life.

In Remembrance of My Grandfather

Hayden Floyd
Rock Springs Middle School, Grade 7

I remember the look of joy on your face when I visited you.

And the warmth that flowed through you as you smiled.

I remember the happiness every Christmas, sitting in your chair, ever so proudly.

And the shirt that said, "I don't want to, I don't have to, you can't make me, I'm retired," that you wore almost every visit.

I remember when you said I was your best buddy.

And I remember the dread when you were in the hospital.

I remember the overflowing happiness when you started to recover.

And the overwhelming sadness when they said you put up a fight and they did all they could.

I remember walking into the room where I would last see you, lying there so calm, serene, and having no regrets.

And I will always remember the last thing I said to you, "I was honored to be your best buddy."

My Baby Sister

Hannah Tucker
Cedar Grove Elementary School, Grade 1

I hope I have a baby sister one day. I will name her Abigail. We will play together. We will play hide-and-go-seek. I will read to her. I will help her when she needs help. I will love her very much and be the best big sister ever.

My Cousin Devin

Triston Wise
Cedar Grove Elementary School, Grade 4

My cousin Devin and I are best friends. We are each other's biggest treasures. We like to climb. Once we climbed on top of a shed. It was fun. It is also fun when we battled with sticks. I hit him on the right, and he struck me on the left side. We did everything together until I moved to Tennessee. We rode bikes, went to lunch, went to theme parks, climbed, and watched TV together. We also did our homework together. Homework is boring to death. But, we could help each other out if we had trouble. Devin and I are twins (we look just alike). Now that I am in Tennessee, I only get to see Devin at school breaks. I miss everything about him.

Little Brother

James Truett
Thurman Francis Arts Academy, Grade 4

Dear Little Brother,

You have taken all the attention away from me and made me not an only child. When

you wake me up in the middle of the night, I want to give you back, but I can't.

Although when you smile, you make me happy especially when you say "goo."

I love you little brother,

James

A Sad Ending

Alexa Massar
Thurman Francis Arts Academy, Grade 4

One memory that I have is when my Grandpa died in April. He died from cancer. From that day on, I always started crying. On Christmas I thought of something where I would always see him. I thought that we could make an ornament with his picture on it. So now, every Christmas, I will see him!

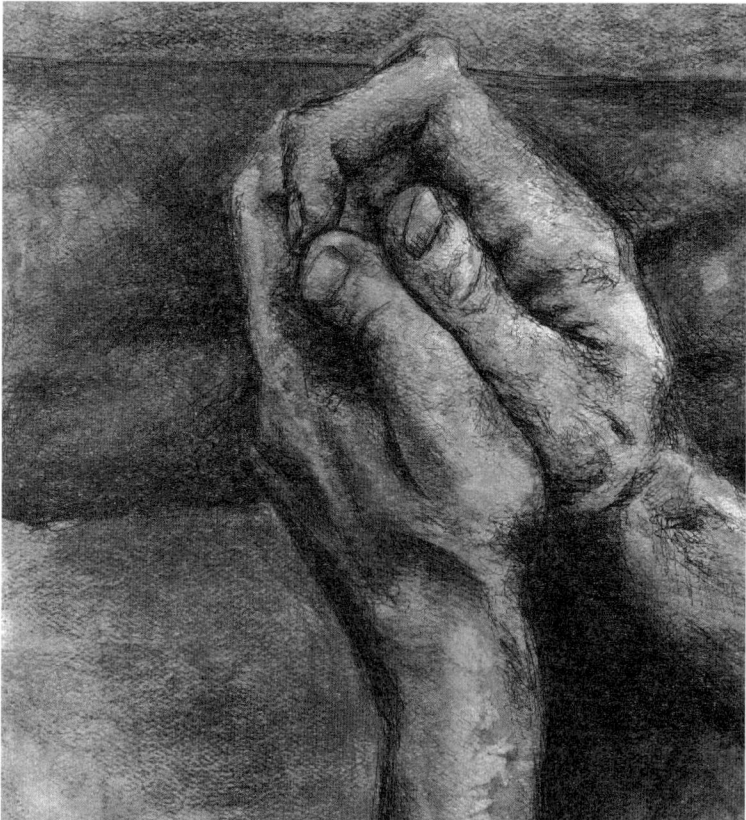

Nancy Sayavong, Riverdale High School, Grade 10

Life Treasures

Dajiah Platt
Cedar Grove Elementary School, Grade 4

The two things I treasure the most are my parents and my dog. If I didn't have them in my life then I would be a complete lunatic.

The reason my parents are one of the best treasures I could ever have is because I have so much to thank them for. They spend most of their good earned money that they make mostly on me or my brother. It makes me feel really good that they would do that.

The reason my dog is one of my treasure is because she is so important to me. She is like a sister to me. She is very playful and she is also one of the weirdest dogs I have ever laid eyes on.

My parents and dog mean more than air to me. I love them very much. They are my treasures.

My Story

Kyndall Brooks
Thurman Francis Arts Academy, Grade 4

When my brother was going to be born in just a couple of days, I got the flu. I missed school for about two weeks. My mom had to go to the hospital the day after we found out I had the flu. I had different people coming to my house to watch me. The day after my brother was born, we found out my dad had the flu, also. When my mom came home from the hospital, my cousin was still over, giving me a bath. My mom yelled, "It's a boy!" I was so happy, but the bad part was I couldn't hold my brother for four days! When I did get to hold him, I had to wear a mask. It turned out to be okay. Now I can play with my brother all I want!

Preschool

Shelby Morrison
Thurman Francis Arts Academy, Grade 4

On one Wednesday, my mom went to work.
She is the best preschool teacher.
And after school, we went to church,
And we all listened to the preacher.

But on that Wednesday
My mom had quite a day,
So when she came home
She got down on her knees to pray.

So after that
She had a little snack,
She didn't know what to choose
So she had a little pudding pack.

She told me how her day had gone,
She told me how her day had gone;
So I looked up at her lovingly, and said,
I really, really love you Mom!

My Treasure

Luis Paz
Smyrna West Alternative School, Grade 8

Treasure is gold
Treasure is nice
I have a treasure that I love with all my life.
That treasure is better than gold
It's nicer than a rainbow
That treasure is my baby sis.

Helping My Mom and Dad

Peyton Pope
Smyrna Primary School, Grade 1

I love helping my mom and dad. My job is to take the trash out. It really stinks bad. It is disgusting! Mom and Dad are lucky to have me as their son. They are happy when I help them.

My New Baby Sister

Jaelen Phillips
Blackman Elementary School, Grade 2

My mom had a baby yesterday. My brother, dad, and I went to see the baby. I got to hold her. She was not awake when we got there. We stopped and got some Krispy Kreme doughnuts. I was glad I got to see my baby sister, Alexandria. She is coming home today.

My Treasure

Devin West
Blackman Elementary School, Grade 3

My mom is:
Outstanding
Trusting
Honest
Exciting
Respectful

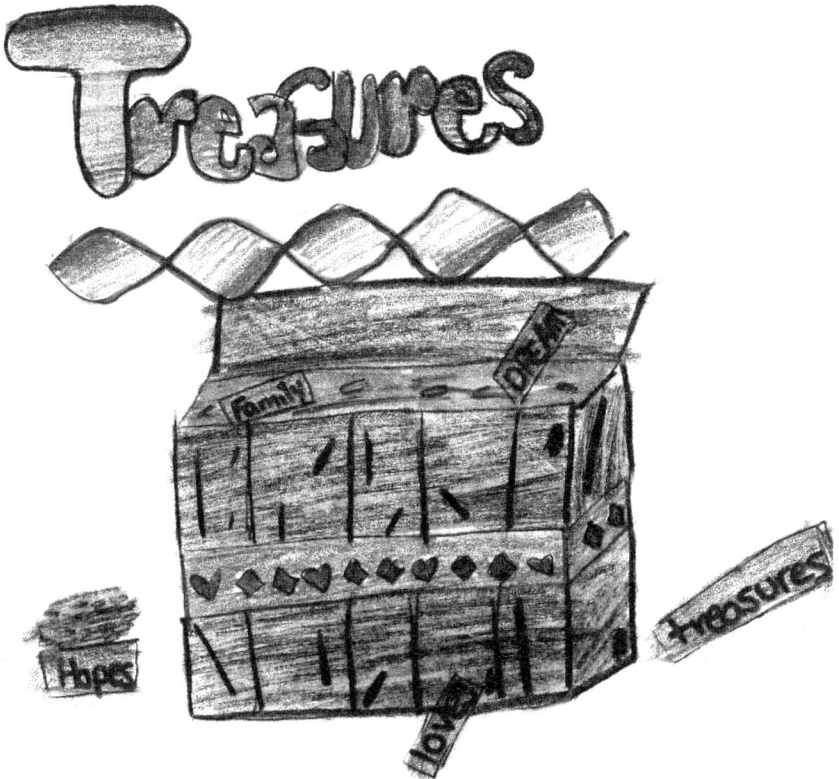

Kara Windrow, Eagleville School, Grade 6

Name Poem

Katelyn Meredith Stringer
Smyrna High School, Grade 10

My name is Katelyn Meredith Stringer.

Katelyn sounds happy and cheerful as if little leprechauns are dancing around you as you say it. After all, it is Gaelic, meaning "pure." Like a pristine waterfall that flows through a green valley that has never been toughed by man, Katelyn flows off the tongue. Or it could be like a Pūr water dispenser pouring clean pure water into a little Dixie cup. Whatever works.

Meredith is like the brave king who fights for the freedom of his people, then protects them from harm during a long and prosperous reign. This chivalrous king must have lived in Wales since the name is Welsh. Or it could be like the little brown-haired girl who rules the Welch's juice empire. (Is her name Meredith?) Either way, the kingdom is prosperous. No wonder Meredith means "great ruler."

Every noble name needs an even nobler last name. Unfortunately, this is not one of them. The name "Stringer" comes from the English lads who decided to name themselves after their occupation. A stringer was a maker of string. What kind of string, we may never know. Perhaps it was shoestrings or bowstrings or the little strings that always come on the green beans. Maybe it is better that we don't know.

Between the dancing leprechauns, the pureness of clean water, and the valiant ruler, my name gives me quite a lot to live up to. Alas, my lowly string-making last name not so much. Yet, there is still hope for my name; I shall get a new last name later in life. But, until then, I am left with Katelyn Meredith Stringer, the purely great ruler of the string-making empire!

My Treasure
Ashley Jaco
Oakland High School, Grade 12

Dear Granny,
      I love you so much! You have taught me so much and you have always been there for me. Through my hard times, when I was falling down, you were there to pick me up. You watched me through my good times as well. I love you, Granny. You are my knight in shining armor. You are my rock. For all of this, you will forever be my treasure.

I love you!
Ashley

Food Writing
Prerna Gupta
Smyrna High School, Grade 10

      One of my favorite foods is my grandmother's crushed *laddoo*. A *laddoo* is a type of sweet Indian dish in the shape of a sphere. My grandmother makes this for me every time I visit India, so I only get to have it about every two years. My mother can't reach the perfection and level of deliciousness as my grandmother in this dish, so she doesn't make it very often. Only my grandmother knows <u>exactly</u> what to include, what not to include, and how to make it, so learning the secret formula of this delectable dish is not easy.
      Crushed *laddoo* is a soft, yet deliciously sweet, tan-colored dish that makes your mouth water and melts in your mouth like butter in a microwave. It leaves a taste sensation so big that you realize you cannot live the rest of your life without it. The sweetness of it is not overwhelming, but rather at a satisfying level that leaves you craving for more. The texture of this dish is of a subtle grainy type, almost like powder. Whenever it is being made in my grandmother's old and experienced kitchen, the bold, yet pleasing, aroma fills the whole house up (and may I say, it's a pretty big house). Wherever you would go, the scent would follow you and constantly remind you of my grandmother's famous *laddoos*.

My Greatest Treasure
Deeyon Kamtarin
Oakland High School, Grade 12

Treasure, it can be many different things that mean the most to us; for me; it is my family. Without my family I would not be able to overcome some of the things that I have been through. They give me support, love, and encouragement; three very significant characteristics that aid in success. I am very thankful for them and their attitudes towards me. I believe with them, I can achieve and overcome anything.

My Grandfather

Amber Buck
Blackman Elementary School, Grade 5

My Grandfather is cool. On rainy day, we'll play in the rain. He'll slip on my shoes so my toes will be dry. He'll also put on my coat so I won't be soaked. We'll splish and splash all day and say, "Oh rainy, oh rainy days." When the day is done we'll take a nap. Oh yes, my grandfather.

Grandmother

Cameron Tynes
Blackman Elementary School, Grade 4

Gives me ice cream.
Rides with me to the doctor.
After school, picks me up.
Never do I not have fun with her.
Doesn't get mad.
Master at having fun.
Often makes us cookies.
The best grandmother ever.
Have a giant bed.
Everyone likes her.
Roses are her favorite flower.

Special Family Times

Noah Dunn
Walter Hill Elementary School, Pre-Kindergarten

My most favorite time is Mommy playing with me.

Untouchable and Glamorous

Reissa Portillo
Smyrna Middle School, Grade 7

I remember the smell of my mom's perfume when she went out for a special event.
She smelled like vanilla sugar all the time.
She always wore this white dress that looked like snow.

I remember her saying, "I love you guys,"
Giving us hugs and kisses on the cheek.

I remember the times she always said, "No," if I asked to come.

She always looked untouchable and glamorous.

My Treasures

Carmen Perry
Blackman Elementary School, Grade 1

My mom and dad are my treasures.

My Grandpa Is My Loved One

Solomon Masarweh
Barfield Elementary School, Grade 4

My grandpa is my loved one, because he has lung cancer. I went there two weeks ago to check up on him. While we were there, I got to go to his hospital. When we went inside, we had to have a pass, and we did. So we went up to the third floor and went to the room 307.

After a few hours, we left and went to my mom's sister's house and we went to sleep. The next day, I made a card for him. He loved it, and started to cry. He said, "I love you, too." The next day, he told us he will sell the house and come to Tennessee. A couple of hours later we came back to Tennessee.

My Special Family

Josselyn Lopez
Walter Hill Elementary School, Pre-Kindergarten

The most special time with my family is camping and going on a picnic.

My Brother

Jordan Fullerton
Wilson Elementary School, Grade 5

My brother is the coolest person I know.
Sometimes, though, I want him to go.
He loves the game of Halo 3,
But not as much as he loves me.

Baseball is his game,
And he thinks soccer is very lame.
There are times we fight,
But in the end, I love him with all my might.

My brother is the coolest person I know.
My love for him will always grow.
He is my hero 'til the end.
I know my heart he will always mend.

My Family

Mark Johnson
Thurman Francis Arts Academy, Grade 5

I have a great family,
I know that is true.
For without my family,
I don't know what to do.

We play games together,
And take many trips.
We love to take pictures,
And watch video clips.

We swim and fish,
But this is my plea.
Grab a controller,
And let's play the Wii.

The Upside-Down Roller Coaster Ride

James McCandless
Walter Hill Elementary School, Pre-Kindergarten

The most special time I had with my family was going on the roller coaster and we went upside down. We went fast and I holded on. You have to make a circle because it goes around.

My Daddy

Kaylei Estes
Wilson Elementary School, Kindergarten

I love my daddy! He is in the Army. He is in Baghdad. He is fighting for our country. He is tired. He doesn't get to sleep much and he works a lot. He called me and said he loves me! I miss him!

My Mom Is Special

Teagan Layhew
Walter Hill Elementary School, Pre-Kindergarten

My Mommy is special because she gave me her lipstick and it's mine now.

Mammoth Cave

Jordan Slone
Wilson Elementary School, Kindergarten

I love to go to Mammoth Cave with my family. I like to get rocks there and look at them. I love going into the cave and looking at all of the stuff. I love spending time with my family.

Treasured Memories

Caleb Smith
Wilson Elementary School, Grade 2

I can remember that Christmas when my dad and I threw snowballs at my mom. After that we made snow angels. Then Mom, Dad, and I built a snowman. Then we all went inside to warm up. We were happy sitting together.

My Papa

Taylor Fitzpatrick
Blackman Middle School, Grade 7

I sprint as fast as I can to jump into my papa's arms. I'm ready to play in the dirt so that I can get as filthy as a chimney sweep. Papa's thin, gray hair, or at least what is left of it, looks better than ever. His wrinkly face sparkles as he sees me approaching. His entire body is as wrinkly as a prune. His plaid long-sleeved shirt covers his arms while his overalls overlap them. I jump into his arms, and he squeezes me like I am a washrag being wrung out. He is a serene, gentle man.

My great-grandfather was an inspiration to me. He always sparkled and shined in the hardest of times. He had an amazing garden about three feet tall. It always was my playground, a place where I always played in the dirt it contained. From the spectacular flowers to the delicious green beans, it was my own retreat. My papa was also a fisherman. He was always at the local lake catching big fish. I don't ever remember visiting his home without enjoying a scrumptious fish. I loved my papa and his kind and loving nature.

As we leave his home, I look out the back window of the car and wave goodbye to my papa. I'll miss his warm and inviting trailer home. I'll miss his red, squishy tomatoes. I'll miss my papa.

Family Treasure

Jasmine Christian
Wilson Elementary School, Grade 2

My treasure is my family because they love me. I love them, too. We play games. We eat dinner together. I play with my brother and sister. I thank God because he made my family.

My Mama, My Treasure

Greer Kimbell
Blackman Middle School, Grade 7

Today, I got loaded with homework, busted my knee when I tripped in the hallway, and to top it all off, I have a fiddle lesson tonight that I haven't even prepared for. Once the bus finally drops me off at my house half an hour late, I ponderously walk across my front yard, dreading the homework weighing my backpack down. I slam my door open and drag my backpack inside, throwing it across the floor. Just as I'm about to go up to my room, I suddenly realize there's someone else in the room. I spin around and there in the red chair is my mama, beaming at me with a big smile on her face. I immediately feel an enormous pressure lifted off my shoulders, for I know my mama will comfort and help me to conquer my problems. Whether I need advice about fiddle stuff or school, my mama is always there to support me all the way. Now the thought of all that homework doesn't damper my spirits at all! My mama is a really helpful person.

Whenever I'm down or hurt, my mama is always there to comfort me. I absolutely love her chocolate oatmeal cookies, and when she makes them for me I feel loved and comforted. Even though I probably aggravate my mama all of the time, she still calls me her "Sweet Pea" and rubs my back in the mornings. She is so kind and selfless that I want to improve how I act.

My mama always thinks of others besides herself. She cooks breakfast for my sister and me, packs my lunch, makes my bed, cleans the house, and always gets me new clothes instead of getting herself some. I wonder how she does it all sometimes, but I know nothing is impossible for my super mom! I know she gets worn out sometimes, but she still does generous and kind things for my whole family. My mama sets a good example for others with her gentle ways, and I love her for it!

Tonight as I go to bed, I feel carefree and happy. Right when I got home from school, my mama set to work helping me with my homework and planning things out so I had enough time to practice for my fiddle lesson. As if that wasn't enough, my mama gingerly bandaged my knee and gave me some of my favorite cookies. When I think about all these things my mama does for me whenever I need her, I realize how much I love and treasure her. I know that if a time comes that I feel alone in this world, my wonderful mama will always be there by my side, ready to do whatever she can to help me endure any hardship that comes my way. I treasure many things, but my unique mama is definitely at the very top of my list!

My Treasure
Gabe Morris
Walter Hill Elementary School, Grade 2

I have a little brother
and I play with him a lot.
His name is Garrett Lynn
and he's the only one I've got.

When I didn't have a brother
sometimes I got bored.
Now I help him with some things
like opening the door.

Sometimes he gets mad
because I'm bigger than he is.
We all laugh at him a lot
He's funnier than any other kid.

Body of Love
Kendric Dartis
Oakland High School, Grade 10

The arm wraps soft love around me,
The hand picks me up with comfort when I'm down.
The heart longs to love and to nurture.
The head is beauty and integrity.
Granny's entire being is love.

Letter to My Daddy

Kayelen Batey
Eagleville School, Grade 3

Dear Daddy,

My memories with you are my treasure. I didn't get to have you very long to make very many memories, but there are a few things I do remember.

I remember waiting at the door when I heard your car coming up the driveway. You usually would be coming home from work. I would run to the door, and you would open the door and pick me up while giving me a kiss. I also remember on my second Christmas you gave me a puppy that I named Coa-coa. You had put a red bow around his neck, which he had almost torn off. Coa-coa will be seven years old this Christmas.

One of my last memories with you is when we went to the beach the first time. You and I took a walk on the beach. The waves would crash into me knocking me down, but, you would catch me so I wouldn't fall down into the sand.

I only had a little bit of time with you, although some other people had more. The time I had with you is a treasure to me because in life you have only one daddy. I even had my one special name for you, Da. I miss you Daddy.

> Love,
> Kayelen

My Grandfather – a Great American Soldier

Sarah Williams
Walter Hill Elementary School, Grade 3

America is one of the best places a person can live! All of the soldiers have helped us a lot. My grandfather was in the Army for thirty years. He traveled all the way around the world. He lost all of his teeth but one. He got hurt really, really, very bad. Now he can't drive or hear. But I still love him just the way he is now. I love you just the same. "Da" you rock!

My Dad

Keith Gregory
Walter Hill Elementary School, Grade 2

My special treasure is my Dad. He is in the Army. He fights for our country. He has to stay in Iraq for a year. He is a volunteer firefighter, too. He helps me practice baseball at home and takes me to my baseball games. I like it when we play in the pool together. He takes me to get a haircut when I need it. I like it when he takes me out to eat. He picks us up from school when he is here. I watch T.V. with him. He helps me do my homework. My dad grew up in North Carolina. I was born in North Carolina, too. My Dad's middle name is my first name. He is the best Dad. I miss my Dad and I love him.

Treasures

Savannah Tanksley
Christiana Elementary School, Grade 5

Have you ever treasured something dear to the heart?
Like a day when someone or something comes home to you?
My brother came home after he graduated Marine boot camp.
He only got to stay for ten days, but they were the best days of my life.
He is still in service, and…
                    I'm so proud of him!

My Big Brother

Savannah Stevens
Walter Hill Elementary School, Grade 2

I want to tell you about my big brother, Samuel. He fixes me Eggos and cinnamon toast. We like to ride our dirt bikes together. Sometimes he helps me with my homework. These are things we do together!

My Dad Is My Treasure

Rene Ross
Walter Hill Elementary School, Grade 2

My daddy is my treasure. He served my country for me.
He works hard for his family. He takes me to the barn. He takes me horseback riding. He loves me very much. I love him more. I am Daddy's little cowgirl. God gave me a special treasure.

My Stepdad

Christian Mitchell
Walter Hill Elementary School, Grade 2

My stepdad is special to me. He is special to me because he took me in when my real dad gave me up. Since then, I have lived with my mom and stepdad. He has treated me like a daughter. Jeremy Lampley is a really good man.

My Dad

Angelica Cole
Christiana Elementary School, Grade 5

My dad is very special to me; he's a treasure to the soul.

He was always by my side through thick and thin. We did some special things together, before he passed away. He taught me how to shoot a gun and showed me how to run and run. He said he could calm the storm, even when the days were warm.
He taught me how to play the game of chess and after we finished playing, my room was in such a mess!

My dad is very special to me; he's a treasure to the soul.

I Treasure

Brianna Field
Christiana Elementary School, Grade 5

I treasure my papa
The laughs we share
The gifts he brings
His Harley he owns
I treasure my papa

I treasure my papa
The things he does
The pictures we take
The time we spend together
I treasure my Papa

I treasure my papa
The joy he brings
How hard he works
The love he spreads
I treasure my papa

Treasures

Aislyn Welch
McFadden School of Excellence, Grade 2

I treasure my family because they are so nice.
My family is fantastic.
I treasure them because of the love we share.
We hold each other when we are sad or scared.
I treasure my family because we play together.
Family is the best treasure a person can have.

I Remember My Sister

Keaton Shearron
Oakland High School, Grade 11

I remember when we stayed up late giggling about little secrets
That wouldn't let us go to sleep…

I remember when we became princesses
Just by dancing on Daddy's feet…

I remember when we discovered new worlds
Underneath blankets that became sails on couch-cushion boats…

I remember when we put on Mom's old clothes
And they turned us into glamorous women…

I remember when you became the strong one and held my hand
When we walked into my first day of school…

I remember when we became gourmet chefs just by cracking an egg into a bowl
While mom secretly picked out the eggshells…

I remember when we played Barbies way too long
Wanting deep down to stay little girls…

I remember when you grew up and I still wanted my dolls
You taught me how to relate in a more grown-up way…

I remember when you first had a broken heart
It became my broken heart too…

A remember how a parking lot became the first real distance that had ever
   been between us
As I stood saying goodbye to you and even to a part of myself…

I remember all the hours and days of our childhood
When the word "sister" became so much more than a word.

My Treasure, My Family

Nausheen Qureshi
Siegel Middle School, Grade 7

Everyone has a treasure, which is something they hold dear;
It helps them remember memories whether they be about times of joy or despair;
It means more to them than gold, for nothing could make them part with it;
It can be an item, memory, or dream;
If you part with it, you would not be yourself;
My treasure would be my family, which completes me;
They are like a blanket that shelters me from winter's cold;
Or a home that protects me from this harsh world;
No matter where I am, they are always there to my rescue;
My treasure, my world, my FAMILY!

Last Gift

Jessica Lamanda Pew
Eagleville School, Grade 5

My Bible is
Out of shape,
It has ripped edges,
Dull colors,
Words of wisdom,
And pictures of Jesus.

My Bible is
Smooth in some places,
And rough in others,
It feels like silk on the inside,
While tethered on the cover.

My Bible is
Warm, loving, and sweet
Just like Uncle Todd
Whom I think of every week.

Mama Harlie

Isaac Haley
Eagleville School, Grade 6

Though she never saw me
She loved me just the same.
She didn't know if I was a boy or a girl
She didn't know my name.

She waited with excitement
For that special day.
But before I could get there
She suddenly passed away.

You see, Mama Harlie
Now lives in heaven and watches over me.
I know since I'm a Christian
One day, together we will be.

My Mom

Rebecca Webb
Central Middle School, Grade 7

First is my mom's beauty,
Like the glistening dew of dawn,
Then it's like the moonlit sky,
As it begins to glow,
To have to say,
That she is as radiant as the stars,
And that I will love her forever more,
And now I am glad to say,
That this is why,
I treasure her this way.

Treasures

Zackery Smith
Siegel Middle School, Grade 7

Family is like a flower;
It has many parts,
Many petals,
Many members.
Combined, it is beauty.
A stem for support and growth,
The heritage of a family,
Simple and full of splendor,
Love so pure and tender.
Family
A flower.

In Memory of My Grandmother

Dylan Paty
Buchanan Elementary School, Grade 5

A million times we needed you
A million times we cried
If only my love could have saved you
You never would have died
Your two loving eyes closed to rest
But in our heart
We knew that God took the best.

My Family

Lauren Piety
Riverdale High School, Grade 12

They give me comfort that gold and silver cannot.
Diamonds and jewels could never love me as they do.
I could live in mansions, or castles with towers to the sky,
But it would never compare to the home they provided.
You could give me treasure to fill one million rooms,
But nothing will mean more to me than they do,
My family.

Treasures of the Heart

Josh Harris
Eagleville School, Grade 6

When you think of treasure you might think
Gold, diamonds, sapphires, and all things nice.
But when I think of treasures,
I think family, friends, and the way Grandpa winks
At me to show his love
Or on my birthday,
When Mom makes blueberry pancakes.
That's what treasures are to me.

Up in the Blue

Meghan Rice
Thurman Francis Arts Academy, Grade 7

Reminiscing about that day brings tears of pain to my eyes
Sometimes this feeling gets to me; it makes me want to cry

I stare at your pictures,
I see you staring back,
But every time I try to remember, my memory fades to black.

I wish I could remember
Who you truly were,
But every time I do, it all seems like a blur

I'd do anything to be with you,
But I know I must go on.
It's sad you're not here with me,
But I know you're exactly where you belong.

They say heaven is peaceful,
And a place far from here
Are these rumors true, Grandpa?
Is it humble; is it dear?

I miss you tremendously,
But I'm happy for you too.
I hope to see you soon,
Up there in the blue.

Treasure

Morgan Goodman
Blackman Elementary School, Grade 3

I have lots of treasures—a teacher, a friend, maybe even a game—but I have a greater treasure, my mom and dad. They've always been there. When I'm scared they help me. They care about me, keep me safe, and teach me almost everything! I might aggravate them (sometimes). I love my mom and dad. If I didn't have them, I probably wouldn't last long. What would I eat? Where would I live? We've had fun every year. At Christmas, we go to a place called Santa Village! Every summer we go to the beach! I love my mom and dad.

India, My Home

Sidhartha Sinha
Smyrna High School, Grade 9

India, a memory in the past,
imprinted within me to forever last.

Spending time with family, always great,
laughing, playing, talking, enjoying, things we appreciate.

All the places and sites to see,
the journeys, constantly filled with fun and glee.

Wherever I go, wherever I roam,
I'll always remember, India's my home.

Teddy

Bobby Shuey
Blackman Elementary School, Grade 3

Teddy is my treasure. I picked him for Valentine's Day for my grandpa. I really liked him, so I gave him to my grandpa. My grandpa got sick and died a couple of weeks later after Valentine's Day. My grandma gave me Teddy. My grandma told me that my grandpa gave it to me when he died.

Teddy is pink and white. He has a ribbon around his neck, and he's striped. I named him Teddy because my grandpa's nickname was Teddy.

My Grandfather

Emily Wood
Smyrna High School, Grade 9

I think back to when he used to be around
His laughter would always fill the room with warmth
His smile could brighten up anyone's day
He always had that look in his eye
That reassured you that everything would be okay
His presence could fill anyone up with joy
His words were both wise and kind
He never once showed fear
Because he was strong in both heart and mind
My grandfather was a agreat man
His love was genuine and unique
His heart was pure as gold
He will always live in my heart
With these memories I treasure and hold

My Twin?

Khendal Lillard
Eagleville School, Grade 12

My Twin?
This guy is my twin? How could this be?
For I am shorter and he is taller than me.
Some say we look alike but I can't tell,
We seem so different, we always fight and yell.
He's tall and so am I, he's skinny but yet I'm fat,
Believe me, ladies, there is nothing wrong with that.
For I am charming, witty, and bold,
He is my total opposite truth be told.
Although we are different we are also alike.
That is something I have learned in life.
We both can sing, dance, and rap.
We can do any dance, (but we've never tried tap).
We are both athletic; we excel in sports.
When I was injured my brother carried the torch.
We both love to win and hate being defeated.
When we compete against each other things get pretty heated.
Yes we talk trash but somehow we work it out.
After all, isn't that what family is all about?
Although mother has confirmed this fact time and time again
I still find myself asking…
How could this dude be my twin?

145

Legacy

Cody Lachance
Christiana Middle School, Grade 7

Two weeks ago was the saddest day for me
Very unexpectedly, at 38, my dad died.
The only wish I have left is to bring my dad back to life,
Even if it's only in a dream.
All the good times I had with my dad will never be forgotten.
The secrets between Dad, my brother, and I will never be told.
The pictures of my dad will be cherished forever.
My brother and I are legacies of our father.

My Treasure

Ben Nguyen
Christiana Middle School, Grade 8

My family is my treasure
Their problems worked out
With cooperation in the kitchen
The football game on the front lawn
The joy of being here
The same differences
My family has come
They are my treasure

My Big Sister

Amelia Zeller
Walter Hill Elementary School, Grade 4

My big sister is twelve. I am eight. She was born in 1995. I was born in 1998. I love my sister even though we fight A LOT!! She has saved my life! We were at my aunt's pool and I got into the six foot-deep end when I was three. I was starting to go to the bottom, when I couldn't come back up and she jumped in and saved my life. Now that she is older it takes her forever to put on her make up and everything in the mornings. Sometimes I tell her I hate her; I never mean it though. Another thing I don't like about her growing up is she fights with my parents all the time. I never get to talk to her anymore because she always has her stinking ipod in her ears. I try talking to her but then all she says is "What?" and it gets annoying. But the point is she's my sister and I lover her, and I look up to her.

Mom

Erika Cripps
Christiana Middle School, Grade 8

Mixture of food she cooks
Her voice saying, "I love you"
The warmth as she smiles
Her sweetness in the air
My treasure
Mom

Grandpa Dewey

Sarah Hoff
Blackman Middle School, Grade 8

The memories of Grandpa Dewey
Are my only true treasures.
Fishing at the lake up in Big Sandy,
Riding his Kawasaki down the
Old road by the river.

His smile and his laugh
As he chuckled at me, and
The way he used to whisper
Sweet nothings in my ear.
My memories of Grandpa Dewey
Are my only true treasures.

Even though he's gone home now,
I know he never left me.
The memories I have of him
Will stick with me forever.
My Grandpa Dewey is a true treasure.

I Love Him

Katie Gray
Stewarts Creek Middle School, Grade 6

My daddy died four years ago.
We did everything together.
We would even play with a feather.
I wish he was back here to say
He loved me every second of the day.

147

When You Left

Nayeli Mejia
Smyrna High School, Grade 12

When you left
Mommy was always crying,
We were always
Looking for you.

But now that time passed
You are the one
Looking for us
And the one crying.

When you left
Every night I prayed
For you to come back.

But now that time has passed
You pray for
Us to forgive you.

When you left
I learned to live
Without a father
And to look over my brother.

But now that time has passed
You have learned that
You can't live
Without your family.

A Trip down Kitty Lane

Maria Hernandez
LaVergne High School, Grade 11

I don't know if any of you have ever suffered a loss, but I am willing to bet most of you have. Whether it be the loss of a friend or a really close family member, the pain will always linger in your heart. The same is said of any household pet. You will never know how much they mean to you until they are gone.

I only remember having two pets as such. Both were cats. One particular Himalayan by the name of Teddy was a big part of our little family. My dad brought him into the family near Christmas time in 1995. I was four years old at the time, but I still remember the big brown box in which he was in. He was only a kitten then. A trembling ball of fluff he was at the beginning. Teddy was a stray on the streets of Moses Lake, Washington and was very cautious at first. Later on, he became a bit more mischievous as he grew accustomed to our family.

The next three years of our lives with him were very interesting. He had a knack for getting into trouble even if it was in a humorous situation. He loved to play games like hide-and-seek with my mother. He even chased the dogs from our neighborhood. It was hilarious to see him at it. You know, most animals tend to eat any human food available to them, but not Teddy. The only human food he ate happened to be a bag of Doritos, but only Nacho Cheese Doritos. He was even particular about the brand of cat food he ate.

Needless to say, Teddy was very happy being with us. After those three years, we moved to Tennessee because of our dad. My parents began to grow apart and Teddy became more than just the household cat. He became her companion as my dad finally left my mother. Teddy became her shoulder to cry on the next couple of years to come. He was sensitive to her needs and was always there when she needed somebody to be there. He would kiss her tears away and lay his paw on her shoulder as if to say everything will be okay. My mother began to see someone else a couple of years after that. Teddy was with us until the day he died in January 2005. My brother and I were with my dad for the weekend the day he died. We had no clue that we'd be coming home to a downhearted mother that Sunday afternoon.

My dad left us and fresh tears sprang into her eyes as she turned to each of us for a hug. We sat down and she began to tell us what had happened Friday morning. She had gotten into her car early that morning ready for work. Pulling out of the driveway, the car jerked over an oddly misshapen bump that made her want to stop. She ran into the house after seeing a clump of white and brown fur in front of the car. She ran into her boyfriend, who was on his way to work, and forced him to check out the situation. Teddy, our dear friend, had frozen over night right behind the tire of the car. She had run over the dead Himalayan- her best friend and companion. Before taking my mother to work, her boyfriend scraped the small body from the pavement with a shovel.

We buried him the night we returned. He was tucked away in a white trash bag and placed inside a dull cardboard box, very much like the one he was presented to her in. I still remember my mother's tear-stained face crying mournfully while stroking Teddy through the plastic bag. That was the final good-bye she could give him and the last time she would hold him. She told me later on the next day that she had told her coworkers something the Friday before. She had told them that she didn't know what she would do if her cat died.

Clay Marble

Jonathan Reynolds
Rock Springs Middle School, Grade 6

The thing I treasure most is my clay marble. My cousins Trevor and Ian also have one. The marbles belonged to my great-grandfather. They were his when he was a little boy. They are about 125 years old.

My Uncle Walter had kept them and gave mine to me on my eighth birthday. He wanted to wait until he thought I was old enough to take care of it before he gave it to me. It is very special to me and I want to hand it down to my children one day.

I keep it in a glass case in my room so can see it every day. It is not colorful or shiny like today's marbles. It is a brown color. There are not too many of these marbles left, so I think they would cost a lot if you wanted to buy one, but I would never sell mine!

I Wish

Princess Roshell
Riverdale High School, Grade 10

It was a cold, winter's night. Out upon the streets, people trudged through the snow or rode in their carriages home. Bells were being rung by solicitors and security kept the streets clean from criminals and directed traffic. A small little girl could be seen amongst the crowds of people. She seemed to huddle with herself on the ground, peering over her knees. Her small pig tails had been frozen strands, almost like brittle. While her clothes were like rags, cut up and torn. The girl's face was filthy, stained with dry tears. As those green eyes peaked over her knee caps, she watched as the townsfolk continued to walk by. They either stepped over her or walked around her. It was as if she wasn't there.

So quietly she stood, knowing it was that time when everyone would be in their homes asleep. She began to walk down the empty sidewalk, her body begging for warmth. It was then that she saw a beam of light, dancing out into the streets. Hurrying towards it, she looked into the window, from which the light had come from. Inside, there was a family, feasting on their dinner and laughing together. "I wish I had a family. . ." She mumbled aloud. This caused the head male of the family to stand from his chair. The little girl smiled, it was as if he'd heard her plea and was coming to save her from the dreadful cold air. Pressing her nose against the glass, she awaited eagerly and almost hopefully. It was then that he'd stood there and slowly closed the curtain.

Her vibrant green orbs widened before lowering. Sniffing a bit, she held back those tears that desperately wanted to fall. All she ever wanted was a family or at least to be noticed. Never had she remembered ever having a family or even being loved. After moments of walking, she finally stopped in front of another window, while the flakes slowly began to whiten her dark hair. As she turned her head, she saw yet another family. They seemed to have been putting the star up on their Christmas tree. "I wish I had. . .a family like that." She then breathed against the window pane. Once again, the male of the home came towards the window, but this time he smiled. Walking towards the door, he opened it and gestured her inside. The girl stood there bewildered before accepting. She couldn't believe it, was it really happening? Was her wish coming true? As she worked her way inside, the warm air tickled her cheeks as feeling came back to her toes. Everyone had gathered around her and removed her small jacket and tattered scarf. Blinking, she was finally set it on the shoulders of the male who'd invited her and was given the star. The family surrounding her beckoned her to continue, before she finally put it on top of the tree. Looking around, she watched as they clapped and listened as they cheered. The tears started brimming again until they finally rolled down her cheeks. She was so happy. She finally knew what it was like to have a family and it was the best feeling in the world.

My Treasures

Andy Swann
Christiana Middle School, Grade 8

There are many treasures
Some of great gold
Others of great pride
I treasure how grateful I am
I am very lucky
To be born into my family
They have given me everything
I have shelter
I have food
And most of all
I have love
I treasure all of these things

My Brother

Rachel Wotkievicz
Siegel Middle School, Grade 7

My brother means a lot to me.
Although, sometimes he acts like a crazy bee
I love him tons and tons,
Because when we're together we always have fun.
He gives me love,
I give him care,
And we always, always share
I don't know what I'd do without him...
The light in my heart would be very dim
So I'm very thankful.

My Cousin Samantha

Savannah McCann
Walter Hill Elementary School, Grade 1

My cousin Samantha is mean sometimes.
She is sometimes nice, too.
But one night she was nice because my sister
was being mean to me and Samantha helped
me feel better and that's why I treasure
my cousin, Samantha.

My Sister

Bethany Midgley
Central Middle School, Grade 8

My sister is probably the
Best thing that has ever happened to me.
Even though she is older than I,
We go everywhere with each other.
We were only born fifteen months a part.
She is the best friend that I could ever have.
We tell each other our secret stories:
The happiest and sad
She is there for me when no one else is,
When we get older we will live close and our children
Will be the best of friends.
I love her and always will.
She is a treasure to me.

Grayson

Ashley Beckwith
Riverdale High School, Grade 12

Ten little toes,
One tiny nose,
Moving around everywhere,
Getting into everything,
Walking around in his own world,
Talking in his own language.
Showing me he has his teddy,
Crying, wanting to sleep.
I pick him up and begin to sing.
…He closes his eyes and begins to dream.

A Letter to Poppy and Grammy
Matthew R. Trail
Lascassas Elementary School, Grade 3

Dear Poppy and Grammy,

I miss you so much! I wish that you could have seen Noah. It has been a long time since you went to heaven. I love you very much. I wish you could have stayed longer.

I want to tell you about my life now. We still have a lot of fun going to the mountains. We stay in a log cabin in Pigeon Forge as a family. While we are on vacation in the mountains, we go for car rides in the park.

Last Summer Nathan and I caught our first fish. When I go fishing, I think of you, Poppy. You loved to fish so much.

Grammy, I miss some of your cooking. I especially liked your peanut butter and jelly sandwiches. They were the best!

I love you both and miss you very much!

Your grandson,
Matt

My Favorite Treasure
Christopher Chase
Wilson Elementary School, Grade 3

My favorite treasure is my family. I have a big sister, a mom, and a dad. My sister is really nice to me. She plays games with me and watches movies with me. My dad is really cool. He brings me home fossils, old bottles, and flint rocks. He also plays basketball, and other games with me. My mom is always there to help me, take me places, and to teach me new things. My family loves me so much, and I love them, too. That is why they are my favorite treasures.

Treasure
Alex Moore
Riverdale High School, Grade 12

True treasure to me,
Friend unlike any other,
Only my mother.

My Nanny and I Make Cookies

Jasmine Rucker
Roy Waldron School, Grade 2

"Can we make cookies, Nanny?" I asked. She answered, "Yes!" We made the cookies together. I took the butter and spread it on the pan. Then we put the cookies in the oven. I thought to myself, "You're the best Nanny ever!" The cookies were done soon. They looked good! I got the plates and we sat down together to eat the delicious cookies. They were good! Have you ever thought what treasure really means? "I love you, Nanny!"

Mi Familia

DeAndrae Miller
Riverdale High School, Grade 12

Like God, they're always there
Through thick and thin, together.
Neither silver nor gold
But mi familia I treasure.
They always have my back
Like a great big umbrella
Protecting me from the world.
Like it was dark, stormy weather.
What's life without family?
I suppose it has to be
Misery
Literally
One word, vacancy.

My Family

Quinlan Odom
Blackman Middle School, Grade 8

Words escape me.
I know what my treasures are,
But there are no words to describe them.
None kind enough for my grandma,
None sweet enough for my nephews,
None brave enough for my sister,
None self-sacrificing enough for my mom,
And none loving enough for my dad.
These people are my treasures
And there will never be words grand enough to describe them.

Household Treasures

Jeremy McClain
Riverdale High School, Grade 12

My treasures are in the household.
My father is guidance to do right,
My mother is my comforter when it seems that there is no light,
My sister makes me tingle with her words that are so bright,
My brother gives me humor that makes me laugh all night.
My treasures are in the household.

Siblings Are Treasures

Kayla Sides
Blackman Middle School, Grade 8

She is always there for me,
Through the good times and the bad.
She always makes me joyful,
But never makes me sad.

She's good at keeping secrets,
She never says a peep.
I can put my trust in her,
Even though the only time she's
quiet, is when she's asleep.

She's there to keep me company,
I know she always cares.
Even though her blonde moments,
Can give me quite a scare.

Who is this person so close to my heart?
She is my sister and we will never part.
Whitney Elaine Sides

My Family

Randi Bivens
McFadden School of Excellence, Grade 6

I love my family with all of my heart
I can't imagine us being apart
I hope there will never be a day
Where my love for them will waste away
They're always there for me
I treasure my amazing family.

Treasures
Courtland Parker
Blackman Elementary School, Grade 1

I love my mom and dad and my bruthyr. I love my famule!

Sweet Baby Girl
Morgan Sullivan
Cedar Grove Elementary School, Grade 3

Littlest hands
Softest touch
Prettiest eyes and loved so much
Crying in night
Holding so tight
Seeing her face nice and bright
Looking at her when she sleeps
Makes me cry
When she breathes so deep
Makes me wonder what she'll grow to be
Hopefully she'll be smart like you and me.

Why I'm Thankful
Danielle Annunziato
Blackman Elementary School, Grade 2

I'm thankful for my health and
the food that I eat.
I'm thankful for all the new
friends that I meet.
I'm thankful for my home and
for my family.
But most of all I'm thankful that
I am just me!

Chapter Six
Treasured Memories

I Remember …

Sara Dusenberry
Siegel High School, Grade 11

I Remember that wonderful weekend,
when a small town grew by eighty thousand.
I Remember the early morning drive
and music planned just for it.
I Remember the wide field so crowded with tents
and the grass so high.
I Remember walking into Centeroo,
the meeting place for all the music that was to come.
I Remember the crowds building at the stages
in anticipation for what was to come.
I Remember the confusion had with whether
to go to "This Tent" or "That Tent".
I Remember the loss of hygiene,
so clearly smelled after only the first day.
I Remember the first concerts heard,
the crowds so packed,
but the music so great.
I Remember the heat of the day,
almost suffocating to the point of making you want to leave,
but not quite.
I Remember the music going throughout the night,
watching and listening to it to the point of exhaustion.
I Remember the joy of everyone,
so happy to be there listening to the wondrous sounds.
I Remember the so many different individuals,
all of such different ages.
I Remember that last morning,
the conflicting emotions,
the need to stay and listen,
and the need of a most refreshing and welcomed shower.
I Remember saying good-bye to that weekend of amazing music,
and to that musical refugee camp, Bonnaroo.

Going on Vacation

Steven Brandon
Lascassas Elementary School, Grade 1

When I was 4 years old, I whent to the beach whith my mom and dad. That made me happy becas that was my vacasin and I was at the Behombas. I played in the woter and it was fun playing whith my mom and dad.

Monster Truck Show

Kate Leonard
Lascassas Elementary School, Grade 1

Jon Bradley and I went to a monster truck show. We saw Jerry, the King, Lawlor. Dad bought us a flag. We waved the flag. We saw a truck go over a bunch of broken cars. Jon Bradley's Dad bought us a hot dog. It was fun!

Fishing

Dalton Cantrell
Lascassas Elementary School, Grade 1

When I cot my first fish I liket it because I was two years old. My dad took me fishing and my bait was worms.

I Wish This Would Last for a Lifetime…

Kaitlin Gay
Siegel High School, Grade 11

I remember walking out of the house, inhaling the crisp air.
The breeze softly blew through my
 red curls as the leaves rustled on their branches.
As my dad and I started off to the gazebo at
the park, the leaves crunched beneath our feet.
I remember looking up at him and seeing his
eyes closed with a small grin coming over his face.
I remember thinking how happy I was to be
walking with him, hand in hand.
His hands were
so much bigger than mine.
I remember thinking with him, I was safe; nothing could harm me and butterflies took
over my stomach as I felt that I was walking on cloud 9.
I remember thinking that my innocent seven years of life could not possibly get any
better.
After looking up at him and seeing the joy of experiencing this ideally perfect moment
radiate from his face, I too closed my eyes and smiled because I knew I would treasure
that small moment forever.
I remember my dad looking at me and saying, "Fall is my favorite, Kait."
Because fall was his favorite time of year, it would become mine, as well.
I still get butterflies in my stomach to this day when I step outside and there is that same
soft breeze I felt when I was a young girl.
I still think about that morning when he and I gaited down Parkview Drive in
Burlington, North Carolina, talking about anything and everything.
Though I remember that day so vividly, the one thought that will stick out above the all
others is, "I wish this would last for a lifetime…"

My Visit to the Nashville Zoo

Carly Alsup
Lascassas Elementary School, Grade 1

When I was 5 years old, I was with my Mom. And we went to the Nashvill Zoo! I saw a zebra! The zebre was black and white. It ran fast. I saw a lion too! It was fast to. It was orange and yellow. I saw a snacke! It was green. I felt happe at the zoo. It was a hot day at the zoo.

Where I'm From

McKenzie Gibson
Siegel High School, Grade 9

I am from hot summer days of playing outside
never enough time 'til the sunlight subsides.
Praying this day could last all year,
living in the present and holding it dear.

I am from hours of practice and long days at the field
wiping sweat from my brow, using shin guards as my shield.
This is the way I choose to live my day.
I couldn't imagine life any other way.

I am from building forts and making mud pies
to playing dress up and acting as spies.
This childhood innocence lives with me each day,
even now as a teenager making my way.

I am from pink frilly dresses and Sundays at church.
Never for morals or faith will I search.
Living each day with these thoughts in my head
helps me determine which path I should tread.

I am from organized chaos with people around,
Never a dull moment or tear to be found.
These memories aren't presents or subjects to give.
I will remember these moments as long as I live.

I Caught a Fish

Brayden Pike
Lascassas Elementary School, Grade 1

Once I went fishing. I caught five fish but I got a snag. My dad had to cut the string. It took a lot of time to fix it. Then I caught three fish. My dad was proued of me. Then we went home and we ate the fish.

I Remember My Childhood

Zach Dooley
Siegel High School, Grade 9

I remember my toys I would not share,
A racecar, an army man, a stuffed teddy bear.

I remember almost everyday I would go out and play,
But some day's it would rain and never go away.

I remember never caring about my clothes,
I'd get them muddy then play in the hose.

I remember my mom lifting me above her head,
And I remember my dad carrying me to bed.

I remember the summer ground burning my feet,
Waiting for the ice cream man to come down my street.

I remember the hill that reached to the sky,
And when I was on top I thought I could fly.

I remember when I loved playing in the sand,
I would get a fist full and let it slip through my hand.

But now I don't play with that stuffed teddy bear,
It's sitting in the bottom of my closet somewhere.

And I guess I'm too cool to wait in the street,
And now I never leave home without shoes on my feet.

And it's been a while since I've played in the sand
I guess this is part of becoming a man.

I Like My Horse Paycheck

Kaitlin Taylor
Lascassas Elementary School, Grade 1

I remember when I went to the horse show. I won first plas and that made me happy. My horses name is Paycheck and he walked and ran. I won a blue ribin and mune.

My Best Birthday

Rivers Cook
Lascassas Elementary School, Grade 1

I remember when I was four years old I got a girl horse for my birthday. Her name is Mazy. She is brown, white, and black. She is very sweet. I love her very much.

My Daddy and Me and the Roller Coaster

Bailee Kauffman
Lascassas Elementary School, Grade 1

I can remember when I went to Disney World. And my daddy made me ride a roller coaster. I close my eyes. Then it went around and around. Then I got off. I wanted to ride again.

The Snow Day

Chris Moosekian
David Youree Elementary School, Grade 3

One day in December I work up on a snowy day. I asked my parents if I could go play. They said, "Yes." After that I got dressed and then I went outside. First I made a snowman. After that I made a snowfort. Then I got cold and went inside. I asked my mom if I could have some hot chocolate. She said, "Yes." It was a great snow day in December.

I Remember

Bekah Everhart
Siegel High School, Grade 9

I remember waking up to the sweet smell of my mother's herb garden, and the feel of my sweat on my tiny body from the humid air around.

I remember the loud, fast beating sound of the recess bell, the crunching of children's feet as they race across the gravel. I remember the sound of laughter and screams as the children play tag.

I remember the crisp evening wind brushing my face as I rode my bike to the park downtown. I remember the crackling and grinding sound of my roller blade wheels as I glide down the sidewalk.

I remember the sweet lavender wisteria draping from the pearl white trellis and the swarm of bumble bees surrounding it, the beautiful clear blue water flowing from the fountain, the cement statues lining the walk way of the green way. I remember the weeping willow tree where the game of "hide and go seek" was made popular.

I remember the crisp hum of the church bells at high noon on Sunday afternoons. The smell of fried chicken, turnip greens, and mac and cheese. I remember the cold sweet tea sliding down my dry parched throat.

I remember laughing till I cried with my friend as we played our childish games. I remember the late nights filled with candy, smiles, and the occasional game of "truth or dare." I remember the tears of sadness and longing when the news of our move was announced.

I Remember Mississippi

Fun in the Florida Sun

Alexa Davis
Cedar Grove Elementary School, Grade 1

The Sea-Blaster was so much fun! I also like surfing in the sun. I like to swim in the hotel pool and I like wearing my sunglasses to look cool. Most of all, I like to be in Florida spending time with just my family and me.

A Shattered Heart

Dazmin Dorris
Siegel High School, Grade 9

I remember seeing them sleeping in separate bedrooms.
I remember being confused and saddened at the way they
looked at each other.
I remember never knowing when they were finally going
to divorce.
I remember seeing my brother heartbroken when my dad left.
I remember going to attorney offices with my mom
and signing papers.

I remember the fights over the phone and in-person.
I remember the judge deciding my brother and I were going
to live with our mom.
I remember being the main reason they argued.
I remember thinking it was my fault they divorced.
I remember having no one to talk to about my feelings.
I remember feeling like my world was falling apart.
I remember being put in the middle of a situation I
couldn't control.
I remember all the stress I went through.
I remember my grades failing because I didn't know how
to express my feelings.
I remember wanting to be invisible so people couldn't see that I was hurting.
I remember realizing that there isn't a such thing as a perfect family.
I remember knowing that one chapter of my life had ended and another had begun.

When We Got T-Cup

Sarah Haley
Stewartsboro Elementary School, Grade 3

When I was about five or six years old, we went to see my Uncle Jackie and my Aunt
Ruth for Christmas. We had bought them a puzzle. When you put all of the pieces
together it made a picture of miniature pinscer dogs. They loved it! My Uncle Jackie
breeds miniature pinscers.

Afterwards, we talked a little bit. It was about time to leave. But first, we got to visit
the puppies. My Mom and I were begging for one. Finally, my dad said "yes"!! My
Mom and I were very happy. We named the puppy T-Cup. After that, we drove back to
our house. We still have her and I love T-Cup very much.

Going to Gatlinburg

Michael Boyd
David Youree Elementary School, Grade 3

Hello my name is Michael. One day mom told us that we were going to Gatlinburg. After she told me that I jumped up and down. Then I told my brother and sisters. They were so happy. It took four hours to get there. We played the go carts. It was a blast! After that we went to an Arcade. My favorite game was Wack A Crocodile. Then we had to go back home. I hope we go there again.

My Favorite Vacation

Allyson Campbell
Blackman Elementary School, Grade 2

My favorite vacation was when I went to Myrtle Beach. I was four years old. I went with my mom, dad, papa, nama, Uncle Gegy, Uncle Chris, Aunt Phile, Uncle Jim, and Aunt Alessa. We all stayed in a hotel, condo-house-type thing but I do not know what it was called. I slept in the same room as my Uncle Chris and Uncle Gegy. I slept on the top bunk. We had a pool in the back of the house and I went swimming in the pool. I went shopping with my mom and nama. I went looking for seashells and rocks with my nama. I did a lot of other things with other people, too. I had a lot of fun!

The Best Kind of Treasure

Phillip Parsley
Oakland High School, Grade 12

One cannot measure treasure with wealth or worldly belongings. Instead, the best kinds of treasures are memories that last a lifetime.
Treasure is my first time fishing with my granddad and uncle on Center Hill Lake.
Treasure is summer nights and playing outside and not having a care in the world.
Treasure is holidays at my grandmother's house and the feeling of joy and comfort with my family.
Treasure is jumping off a forty-foot cliff into the lake with my best friend yelling right beside me.
Treasure is kissing the love of my life and knowing she is all I will ever need.
Treasure is playing on the number two ranked baseball team in the entire nation and hitting two homeruns in the same inning.
Treasure is camping out under the stars with my friends and sleeping around a campfire.
Treasure is being baptized and knowing God has a place for me in heaven.
Life is a treasure. The only way to enjoy it is to make memories with those who are most important. After all, memories are the only things we take with us when we go.

These I Treasure Most...

Nicole York
Oakland High School, Grade 12

Memories of childhood
Before innocence was gone
These I treasure most
Memories of friends
Before growing up
These I treasure most.
Memories of family
Before some passed on
These I treasure most.
Memories of love
Before heartbreak occurred
These I treasure most.
Memories.
These are the true treasures of life.

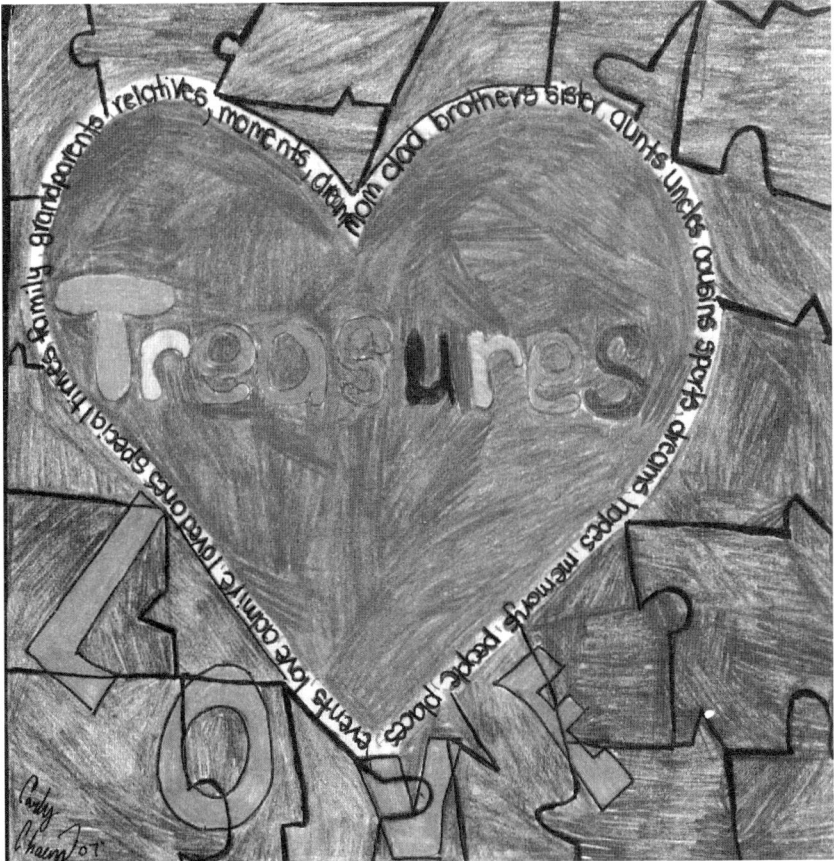

Carly Chavez, Rock Springs Middle School, Grade 7

First Time I Picked Up a Snake

Levi Stone
David Youree Elementary School, Grade 3

The first time I picked up a snake it was the memory of a lifetime. I was three years old when I picked up the snake. It came slithering at me. It snapped! It was all a blur for a minute. Then the snake bit me on the leg. I cried and ran inside to tell my mom. She called the pest control and took me to the hospital. They gave me shots. In a few days, I felt better. I learned to never mess with snakes again.

I Remember

Sarah Kimbrough
Smyrna Middle School, Grade 7

I remember the swings and the merry-go-round

I remember the slides going up and down

I remember my family together on Easter or Halloween,
Playing and talking and making a big scream

I remember my dog Baby; I miss her a lot,
She had fleas and she would itch in one spot

I remember my dad; we always had a ball,
He taught me to get up if ever I fall

I remember my life and all its treasures and tolls,
It is like a bucket for more than one memory to hold.

Under the Knife

Chelsie Augustin
Lascassas Elementary School, Grade 7

It was a warm day in May. I was riding my four-wheeler down a hill when I flipped it. It landed on my left leg, crushing my ankle. I stood up, heard a loud pop, and collapsed. Riding the golf cart, my brother came to my rescue. He flipped the four-wheeler over, and then picked me up and put me in the back of the golf cart. This led to my next adventure.

I was taken back to my grandparents' house. They took one look at my leg and called my dad to come pick me up. It took my dad two hours to get to my grandparents' house. They loaded me up and we started the two-hour drive to Nashville. It was a long, bumpy ride. I was miserable!

When we finally got there, a nurse (my mom) came outside with a wheelchair and took me into a huge waiting room where other patients were waiting for treatment also. I sat in the wheelchair until my mom came and took me to get x-rays. I was glad my mom was at work that day! They took the x-rays and then told me that I was going to have to have surgery.

The next thing I knew they were poking me with needles and IVs. I hated it! After they were done poking me I put on a blue gown. Then they took me into the cold operating room where there were a lot of doctors waiting for me. I got nervous, but the nurses and my mom reassured me. Then they put me to sleep.

When I woke up, my family and friends were around me. My room was full of balloons, cards, and gifts. I lifted the covers to look at my foot. It was wrapped up in a soft cast. With the whole summer ahead of me, I was upset, but my friends and family reassured me that everything would be okay and they would keep me company during the long summer.

Even though I went through surgery and had a cast on for the summer, I still got to swim, drive the golf cart around, and have lots of friends over. Despite going "under the knife," my summer was a blast!

My Auntie's Wedding

Oumie Njie
LaVergne Primary School, Grade 1

One day I went to a wedding. It was my auntie's wedding. When the wedding started, the bridesmaids went first. Then the best man came second. I was the flower girl. I came right before my auntie. I was carrying a basket of flowers that were fake. I was throwing them down all over the floor. I came up the steps. Then the bride and groom got married. My auntie was happy, and I was happy, too!

Memories and Dreams

Megan Foss
Blackman Middle School, Grade 7

M   Magical

E   Exciting

M   Mournful

O   Obnoxious

R   Really sorrowful

I   Irreversible

E   Especially cheerful

S   Special in your heart

D   Daring to dream of anything you want

R   Really great

E   Especially what you want to happen

A   All imagination

M   Magical

S   Secret

The Winter of Snow

Brooks Noland
LaVergne Primary School, Grade 1

One winter day, I was playing in the snow, and I made a snowman. I made snow angels, too. I lay down in the snow and spread my arms and legs out. Then I moved them back and forth. When I went inside, I drank hot chocolate. It made me hot, and I was sweating. I made snowflakes when I cut paper with scissors and made a design. This was a fun day!

State Champion

Caitlin Booker
Rockvale Elementary School, Grade 3

My name is Caitlin Booker, and I am nine years old. I have been a competitive gymnast for two years. I love the competitions, and I get very excited!

The most important meet of the year is our state meet. This year the state meet was at Miller Coliseum in Murfreesboro, Tennessee. I was chosen to be on the All Stars team.

We have four different events that we compete in: bars, beam, floor, and vault. My favorite is beam. I've been told that I'm the best on bars.

I was the first on each event. I was both excited and scared. I had been practicing sixteen hours a week for the big day. I was ready for the competition! I went first on bars and scored a 9.425. Next, I was on a beam, and I didn't wobble a bit. My dismount was incredible! I waited patiently for the judges to flash my score. I scored a 9.45! I was so happy! I only had two events left. Then I was on my floor routine. I scored a 9.4. Last, but certainly not least, was vault. I knew my scores were good and that I needed to finish strong. I finished and scored a 9.325. Now, I had to wait for the final scores.

Everyone gathered for the award ceremony. I felt really good because I knew that I did my best. They started to call names, and mine was last. The state champion on bars was me! Then they said the state champion on beam was me, too! I placed third on floor and vault. They finished the night by announcing the all-around state champion in my age division. That's when I couldn't believe it...they called my name! I was the state champion with an all-around score of 37.6. My coaches and family were very proud of me. I felt proud of me, too. My dad carried me out on his shoulders. I knew I was blessed. I like gymnastics because God gave me the gift to do it.

Why Me

Brittany Mathis
Blackman Middle School, Grade 7

Everyday I say,
"Why me; why did you give me up?
Was I not good enough,
Or did you not love me?"
But the day you gave me up,
I still remember and I cry.
But now I have a family that
loves and cares;
Now I don't need you in my life!!

A Treasured Memory

Rebecca Browning
Eagleville School, Grade 8

The old, brick house with its long, paned windows, stands at the very end of a long street in Gadsden, Alabama. As we drive up the street we see our grandparents walk slowly out of the house to give us hardy welcomes. We walk out onto the porch and hugs and kisses are passed around our little group outside the old door. We go through the door and enter in through the kitchen. A rush of warm air hits me like a cannon ball and the aroma of roast beef and other sweet smelling things pull me to the table. After a nice dinner of laughing, telling stories and jokes that we'd heard time and time again, we'd trudge up the long stairs and take time to look at old photographs on the way. I make my way to one of the cozy little bedrooms and drop my stuff at the edge of the bed, slowly place myself under the soft comforter, and think about how much I've missed this place. Staring up at the ceiling, I drift off to a sweet sleep.

The smell of pancakes, bacon and the sound of laughter awaken me. I lazily put on my clothes and tiptoe down the stairs tying not to wake my parents. Once down in the kitchen, we say good morning and wait till everyone is down there. After we're all together, we say prayers and eat our enormous breakfast. Someone would start up a conversation and everyone starts talking at once; talking about how they're doing in school or how they've been. Finally, we are finished with our breakfast. "Mmmmmm. That was so good! Thank you!" we'd all say. After thanking them for the food and helping clean up, I'd run outside, make my way to their springy trampoline and jump till my legs ached. I'd fall on my back to rest my legs when I hear, "Becca? Do you want to go watch TV and eat ice cream with me?" I nod my reply and race my way towards her and through the door. We'd get some ice cream and make our way down the stairs to where my Great-Grandma used to live. We'd go explore for a while, then settle down on a couch and watch TV.

Not long after we'd hear, "Tori? Becca? Are you down there? Come upstairs, your cousins are here!" As soon as we hear that we are up and running up the stairs to greet our cousins with enthusiastic hellos. The adults go into the living room and grab a chair to talk, while we go outside or upstairs to play until we got tired. Finally, it came time to go. "Mom! Can't we stay for a couple more hours?!" some would whine. "I'm sorry, but we have to get home." Our mom would say pitifully. After we got everything in bags and were all packed up we'd say goodbye and walk out the door. As we walk out to the car, everyone would smile their warm smiles and wave at us saying, "Goodbye! See you soon!" We start to drive down the road and we all turn around in our seats to get a last look at them, and we'd watch the old brick house fade away into the distance.

By the Fire

Josh Crawford
Eagleville School, Grade 8

In the dead of winter, so freezing cold
In the dark of night, black as coal
Around a fire blazing that's so bright

Two brothers sit around that fire
Listening to the crackle of the fire
In the stillness of the dead winter night

They talked and laughed till
The night grew old
But still they talked and laughed
Around that blazing fire

Slowly the blazing fire died down
And they head back toward the house
But never to forget the bonds
They made by that blazing fire

The Misadventures of Snowboarding

Meggan Marvin
Blackman Middle School, Grade 8

I stand outside shivering at my bus stop waiting and waiting. When at a glance I see a snowboarding poster in a window of a neighboring house, I start thinking of a long lost winter and a misguided attempt to snowboard.

As I stepped out of the heated lodge, a slight breeze ruffled my hair. The skiers' echoing cries of "Watch out!" or "Coming through!" disrupted the silence of the valley. Shivers ran down my spine as I thought of what I was getting myself into. The word floated, unwanted, in the front of my mind. Snowboarding. My hand trembled as I reached for the snowboard, a Jolly Roger printed on the front of the board. What an appropriate symbol, for I would probably kill myself trying to attempt this. I traipsed across the powder-like snow to catch my group and set my board binding side down in the multicolored glass gondola. The bright rays of the sun just peaked over the mountaintops as we reached the highest wire of the gondola track. I then looked, terrified, over the edge of the window. A five hundred foot fall awaited the person unlucky enough to fall. We arrived at the platform without a hitch. But for me the real terror was just beginning as I dragged my board across the snow.

My first thought as I strapped my feet into the rock solid binds was " I'm going to kill myself" - an unusually pessimistic outlook for an overly optimistic teenager. I wobbled slightly as I made my way to my feet. The board started to slide down the most infinitesimal hill when all of a sudden I lost whatever little balance I had and landed with a high pitched scream. Then a gloved hand entered my line of sight as my instructor helped me to my feet. What a very ungainly start to what might have been a very comical day to the average boarder.

By lunchtime the loud whoosh of air leaving my lungs was not uncommon. It was the fifty-seventh time I had fallen that day and, if you asked anyone, it only got worse as we headed higher up into the mountains. I had fallen off the chair lift and after picking myself up had started to head towards a small plateau. The board started to slide as I shifted my weight forward and I started to make my way downhill. I gently encouraged the board to turn several times down the small slope. When I reached the plateau I pulled a quick backstop and yelled, "I did it!" Suddenly, I lost my balance and fell flat on my back with a groan. But as with all the other falls, I picked myself up and kept going. You may think it couldn't have gotten any worse...o, but it can and did. I found myself looking at the powdered snow and quickly approaching evergreen trees when my board hit a small patch of ice and lost all grip. Heading away from the jump, I was flying towards a large evergreen. With a dull thud, I collided with the oh so lovely scenery. And with the slightest of movement, I had caused the snow to dislodge from the branches and fall upon my head. I picked myself up while hearing the muffled laughter of two skiers behind me who were doubled over laughing at the sight of my predicament. I quietly gathered a small ball of snow in my hand and with fluid motion threw it. I quickly hopped on my board and headed downhill, ducking as icy missiles flew overhead. At last, I stole quickly into the lodge, and out of sight.

I am brought out of my memories as autumn calls my name, and I see the school bus pulling onto our street. But whenever I remember walking into the lodge, dropping my board dejectedly, pulling off my boots, and sighing, I think of the important lesson I learned that day: trees hurt!

Like a Work of Art

Emilee Wilson
Eagleville School, Grade 8

A treasure can be anything,
Anything you choose.
But there's a kind that's special,
A kind you'll never lose.

Just pick a happy memory,
A simple one will do.
One that's really special,
One that's close to you.

So when you close your eyes,
That memory's bright and clear.
It's something you care for,
Something very dear.

That memory is a treasure,
A little joy for your heart.
Unwritten poetry,
Like a work of art.

Dancing through the Night

Micah Haskins
Blackman Middle School, Grade 7

Some memories linger in your mind forever, never enabling you to let them go because they are attached to your heart, mind, and soul. My memory of my first dance recital is something I cherish dearly, and could not forget even if I tried. From the fitting of the ballet slippers, to the makeup and costumes, and to the moment when the curtain ascends from the stage, I remember it as if it were yesterday.

When I was two years old I asked my mom if I could enroll in dance class. Because I was somewhat clumsy, my mother was a little nervous about it, but nonetheless, fully supportive of my dream. Oh, how exciting was my first ballet shoe fitting! You could smell the new leather of the unbroken shoes as soon as you walked in, and still today I adore that smell. For the next week I lived in those shoes, prancing and leaping around all day until it was physically impossible to do more. Classes started, and I could not have loved it more because being as clumsy as I was, I gained grace and elegance as soon as I stepped onto the dance floor. I was so excited when the week of my dance recital came, and I could not stop thinking or talking about dance.

Preparation the night of my recital was something I adored. My mom curled my platinum blonde hair as I went through my dance repeatedly in my head. Once my head full of ringlets was in a secure beautiful updo, it was time for the makeup. With my iridescent eye shadow, rosy cheeks, and bright red lips, I looked like a beauty queen! My costume was absolutely stunning, and I thought I was the queen of the world in it. Although the pink lace front with the corset in the back was beautiful, my favorite part was the delicate pink tutu fluffed out like a peacock's feathers. I was about to burst with excitement, but my night had only just begun.

When we arrived I had no idea what to think, say, or do. I was awed with the older girls and how beautiful their costumes were, and I longed to be like them when I grew older. We were all rushed backstage and soon we were being told it was our turn to go on, so we filed onto the stage, a sea of empty blackness. Then we got into position while the curtain ascended. My heart was thumping like a drum, and I was afraid the audience might hear it. I was so nervous that it felt like I stood on that stage smiling at a silent audience for an eternity. There was tension in the air, and the light bulbs made us feel like we were standing in the middle of the sun. Then the music began.

Suddenly all of my nerves vanished, and I felt the strangest sensation inside of me. It seemed as if the music was filling me up like a balloon with helium. I felt like I was going to pop. Unlike a balloon, I popped with the passion of dance. It felt as though I was gliding like an angel over the stage and not a care in the world could possibly touch me. My spirit finally ran free on that stage because dance touched my soul. This was complete bliss. To be filled with one hundred percent joy is one of the best feelings in the world because it seems to stop time.

The feeling of complete happiness is something everybody deserves to feel. For me, my first dance recital touched my heart and a person never forgets something like that. Even though my first dance recital was eleven years ago, in my heart I will remain dancing forever.

Memories

Nathan Duke
Oakland High School, Grade 10

Some forgotten, some remembered,
Just like on from last December.
Christmas was a joyful time each year,
Spreading gifts and Christmas cheer.
Eventually memories fade away,
More are made another day.

And soon Spring did come.
This promised that school was almost done.
We always enjoyed the year at this time,
To make more memories, one day to remind.
But eventually memories fade away,
More are made another day.

So then came summer along with its jobs.
Our time was stolen. We felt we were robbed.
The memories that we made with our friends
We hope to do soon again.
But eventually memories fade away,
And more are made another day.

Fall arrived. A year had passed.
And yet some memories did not last
Because eventually memories fade away,
But more will be made another day.
Some forgotten, some remembered.

Our Memories

Jessica Necessary
Blackman High School, Grade 11

When I look back at the time we shared
I remember how much you truly cared
You smiled at me and I got weak in the knees
I'm in awe when I look back on our memories

We've been together for so many years now
It's been so long since the day I made that vow
My heart is overwhelmed with my love for you
Most of the time I can't believe you feel the same way, too!

Memories

Lauren Woods
Rockvale Elementary School, Grade 7

Memories, do they really last forever…
Photos in your mind
Thoughts about your past
They can't be taken away
Although, they may fade
But, always last forever
Remembering; treasuring
Keeping it in your heart

That special person
Never forget
Remember in your mind
How special they really are
Memories that you hold dear
Never let go

Think back to your childhood
Never forget those days;
Playing on the playground
Laughing with your friends

Memories,they're a special thing
Keep them with you
Wherever life takes you

A Trip to the Zoo

Addie Baird
Kittrell Elementary School, Grade 3

One day our class went to the zoo. Cassidy, Nala, my mom, and I got to see all the different animals. My mom got my brother a tiger, and she got me a monkey. I brought binoculars to look at the animals closer. We saw giraffes, monkeys, elephants, tigers, crocodiles, wild dogs, birds, snakes, frogs, fish, insects, and more. We saw a HUGE snake that was long, big, and fat. My mom is scared of snakes, but we still saw them. We even got to pet llamas and donkeys. We got to brush some goats, too. That was great!

My Best Memory
Dakota Williams
Lascassas Elementary School, Grade 4

My best memory is when my papa, my brother J.D., and I go to the creek. I have so much fun. J.D. and I like to find snakes, turtles, frogs, frog eggs, and tadpoles. There are also horses and cows around that we like to watch. We haven't been recently because we haven't seen my papa in a while, but J.D. and I still like to go when we can. I can't wait until the three of us can all go on an adventure to the creek again soon!

St. Jude's
Caleb G. Stewart
Barfield Elementary School, Grade 3

Dear St. Jude's,
  My name is Caleb and my sister Elizabeth has brain cancer. We have been going to St. Jude's since she was four years old. She is ten now and about to have her last chemo treatment. My sister and I have spent a lot of time at your hospital in the last six years. When my mom told us that we wouldn't be going there every week anymore, I was happy and sad at the same time.
  I was sad because I always have fun when I am at St. Jude's. There are always volunteers who like to play with us when we are stuck in the waiting areas. The man in the medicine room waiting area is one of my favorites. He is very good at making paper airplanes. He has made a bunch for my friend Austin and me. Austin is a patient at St. Jude's Hospital and gets chemo on Wednesdays like my sister. We have a lot of fun playing with those planes. I will miss that about being at St. Jude's.
  I was happy because we won't have to miss so much school or drive so much anymore. I was also happy that Elizabeth won't be getting chemo for a while. Mom says no one knows how long it will be before her tumor starts to grow again. Elizabeth is very excited that her hair won't fall out again soon. I was very glad that she won't have to get sick once a week anymore. I hope her tumor doesn't ever grow again, but if it does, I know we will be able to have fun while we ar at St. Jude's.
  Thank you St. Jude's for helping my sister get better and helping us to have fun while we have to be there!

Fires

Chris Moses
Daniel McKee Alternative School, Grade 11

The emergency management truck has just gone by. I didn't want to hear it –"Evacuate Now! The road closes in thirty minutes." I knew that the fires were climbing the canyon walls, but I was shocked to see the flames over the ridge. "Evacuate," they said. I have to pack the car. Why hadn't I packed when the fires started? I had twenty minutes to decide what to take.

I was so nervous I couldn't think of what to grab. I thought to myself for a minute and then went to work. I grabbed all of the essentials including my I.D., driver license, house deeds, money, credit cards, bankcards insurance papers, and meds. The loud town siren woke me from my trance.

Shortly after, I thought, what else do I need? That question was answered quickly. The family jewels and pictures that my mom had gotten. There was an emerald ring that she had gotten from her mom and so on through the generations. I couldn't dare leave that here. So I ran and grabbed and placed it securely in my pocket. The flames were growing closer and closer.

I knew there was something else I should take. Time was running short. The heat and smoke from the fire was affecting my thinking process. The entire house started to smell like the inside of a chimney. The air was getting harder and harder to breath. Flames started to engulf my neighboring house. I thought for a minute and then realized what I was missing. I quickly got started. I grabbed all the material things I would need. I would need a cell phone there was no way I would leave it behind. I needed to stay in touch with my family and friends, not to mention the emergency numbers. I also had to chase my dog Browser down. He wasn't used to all of the commotion. He was frantically jumping up and down. I ran to the car and threw in all of my provisions and treasures, including Browser. He jumped in the front and immediately started to bark when he saw me head back towards the house. I went back and got my electric grill, lots of canned foods, and a set of dry clothes I wanted to be able to change clothes at least once. I also needed blankets; there was no telling where I would be sleeping. There was no time to think; the fires were at my backdoor. I had to get out of there, and I had to do it now!

I leaped out the front door. The flames almost singed my neck hair. Trying to find my car key, I frantically fumbled with my keys. I finally selected the right one. I jumped into my car and sped off. Barely escaping death, my nerves started to settle when the worst sight of my life came upon me. I was too late; the road had closed. I thought I was done for. Just then a fire truck stopped and asked if I needed a ride through the detour. I put all of my essentials in a bag on top of the canned foods I didn't want anyone to know how much I had. I also grabbed Browser and my cell phone. Then I jumped in the passenger seat. I never went back. There was no point. There was nothing left but the destruction of the fires.

Breakfast in Cinderella's Castle

Heather McFarlin
Riverdale High School, Grade 10

We walked into the castle
The food lay out before
The smell was so delicious
The wait I could ignore

There were so many people
Young and old the same
All here for just one purpose
Much more than just a game

We finally heard our name aloud
Above the noise in there
We smiled and walked up to the front
Then climbed the castle stair

Seated by the servant men
And waited on like queens
They called us "Ma'am" and "Misses"
It was better than my dreams

Afterwards there came a sound
And everyone sat still
The princesses came floating in
The silence they did kill

Laughed and smiled all morning long
It was so fun to see
My mother, sisters, cousins, all
The princesses and me!

The Memories

Landry Bobo
Christiana Middle School, Grade 8

The waves crashing into each other
The cool summer breeze
The nice cool mist
The salt in the ocean water
The memories that I will treasure

Summer Camp through My Eyes

Jessica Hildebrandt
Riverdale High School, Grade 11

Rays of sunshine race down to Earth in a blazing frenzy
Kissing the dew placed with perfection on the blades of grass

Laughter fills the air with overwhelming jubilation
Minds cannot comprehend what is to be revealed in the dawning of the new day
But ignorance makes the discovery all the more exquisite and fascinating

Clouds come with rains of confusion
But, even with their haunting shadows
Music is unleashed from the red, fire-filled fingertips
Sailing tenderly down the mystical keys like Earthly winds

Afternoon slumbers renew the tired souls
That have been hammered by the never-ending cycle of agony we call Life

The heart is optimistic and wonders of the undiscovered
New ties yet so strongly made are coming to their breaking points

Even though sad-stricken by the concept of this utopia ending so soon
The soul is overjoyed it was alive to experience
The unexplainable moments of life

Letter

Cayley Foxworthy
Blackman Elementary School, Grade 4

November 5, 2007

Dear Diary,

I want to tell you about my family's special trip to Florida. It was a very warm and beautiful week. It was great!

When we got there, I got to go to the pool. I also got to go to the beach. That was a lot of fun. We saw lots of things at the beach like jellyfish and dolphins. I managed not to get stung by a jellyfish, which was great.

The dolphins were very active. They were jumping out of the water every few minutes. They were also very friendly. I had a great time in Florida.

Until tomorrow,
Cayley

Freshman Treasures

Haley Ferrell
Smyrna High School, Grade 9

Friday night with the crisp fall air,
and the ones I love beside me.
The time I treasured most in life,
seems so far behind me.

Purple and gold filled our stands
while crimson filled the others.
The best of friends beside me
and above me was my mother.

We clapped and cheered and did our best
to show off our school spirit.
We dropped the ball and lost the game,
I guess the players couldn't hear it.

The ending wasn't all that great,
but the night was still amazing.
It's one of those times you'll never forget
in your mind it keeps on playing.

It may be the season or the friend by my side
that won't let my memory forget it,
But when you find the time when everything's right,
make sure you remember and treasure it.

Letter

Bailey Holcomb
Blackman Elementary School, Grade 4

November 5, 2007

Dear Diary,

I have had a lot of trips to many places, but there is one trip that I will never forget. It was during summer break. It was the first time that I went on a trip with everybody in my family! We went to Six Flags in Kentucky. I loved it!

The first thing we went on was the River Rush. It shoots you out of this tunnel onto a lake bed. Next, we went on the bumper cars. My dad bumped every car there. I just chased my sister around the whole time. We went on a lot more rides before we went on this huge roller coaster. Then something really funny happened. The workers realized that I was too small for the ride after I got on. So they had to stop the ride for me to get off. I was disappointed, but still had lots of fun.

Until tomorrow,
Bailey

184

My Dog Precious

Shane Standifur
Smyrna Primary School, Grade 5

It was a cold night, last year, when we realized my dog, Precious, was limping. When my parents examined her they noticed that something was wrong with her leg, but it was too late to head to the doctor. The following morning, she started to cough and was barely walking. We were all trying to decide where to take her, when we heard a yelp from the living room. My other dog, Bailey, had jumped on Precious, wanting to play. I had to take poor Bailey out to the doghouse. We then took Precious to the doctor. The doctor told us that Precious was not going to make it and we should just take her home. I was very sad because I love Precious a lot and I had good memories with her.

The next day, as my father was getting out of work, one of his friends told him to go to a vet in Woodbury. We took her there that same day. This doctor said she might make it, but we had to leave her there for two days. At home Bailey was missing Precious, scratching the door, hoping to get in and snuggle up with Precious.

The day finally arrived, when we had to pick her up. There she was sliding all over the floor. I was so happy that she made it. The doctor said that she had heartworms that were twelve inches long and her leg was healed. The doctor said, "She hasn't been eating well, so give her some biscuits." We took her back home and Bailey was so excited to see Precious back. Today Precious still runs around and wrestles with Bailey. She weighs seventy-five pounds, which is pretty good for a ten-year-old dog.

The First Storm Alone

Tiffany Carlton
Eagleville School, Grade 12

The lightening smells of death
The sky breeds anger
Drops of heaven pound the earth all around me
The wind carries the grain miles from home
Alone under a willow I stand
It's cold and dark, my face heavy with tears
I'm soaking wet, but I don't care
I speak your name and nothing happens
I say it again louder and yet the same response
This is the first storm alone
You're nowhere around I'm truly alone
My heart is broken, I fall to the ground
The sky cracks, the trees sway
And then at once it goes away
The sun comes out
Heaven takes back its drops
And still I'm all alone

Finally...Some Peace

Christopher Cina
Christiana Middle School, Grade 7

I lie in the grass and start to think.
As I am lying here on the ground,
I start to hear dogs barking
I get up and I hear birds singing.
As I am riding my bike, I see little kids.
They are playing together and laughing.
As I am riding and listening, I start to think.
I am thinking about how lovely my childhood wasn't.
Then, I start to think about how lonely I was.
My sad thoughts quickly turn to something else.
Then, again, I think about my childhood,
which was very bad and very sad.
At the same time, I didn't want to think about how bad my life really was.
I became very mad about the way my first two families treated me.
My first family treated me cruelyl; and so did the second, but my third is really kind.
Yes, I now live in a much better home—-they foster kindness in me.
There is no fighting or yelling...there is just peace.
Then, I go into my new home and I lie down.
As I am lying here, I start to think how lucky I really am.
I think about how happy my new family is,
and about the peace that we have here in this house.
Then, I turn on my TV and see the news.
I think about how mean some people are in this world.
For God says to love your enemy and to love your children.
There is complete silence in this house, and I breathe in calmly,
Knowing that I am in a finally in a peaceful home now.

Surprise Birthday Party

Brianna Johnson
Smyrna Primary School, Grade 5

"Surprise," yelled my family as I walked in the door. Today is a special day. It is November 19, 2007, that is my birthday, the second best day of the year. December 25 is the first best day of the year.

Every year my birthdays are always the best birthdays ever, but this year was different. Usually, I only had fifty people at my birthday; however, this year my mom said that I could have as many people as I wanted to. I was so happy and so thankful for my mom.

After we got every thing ready for the party, the guests got there. From there on the party was number one on my list. This birthday is the best one yet. Everybody had a great time, especially me!

I Remember

Seth McCrary
Siegel High School, Grade 9

I remember
Playing in the park
Riding on the teeter totter
Singing happy as a lark,
Rolling in the dirt
After a wild ride
On the slide,
Jumping on the monkey bars
Flying on the swing
Feels like blasting off to Mars,
Or floating on a dream,
Playing tag and hide and seek
With friends is a blast,
Even though I cheat and peek
I still come in last,
Now I must deter
The sun is going down,
It is sad I must leave my wonder
And go back to town.
I remember...

My First Tractor

Jessie Josey
Lascassas Elementary School, Grade 4

My special time was when I got a tractor. I was four years old. It was an orange and black tractor. I drove it all around in the yard. I went to the dirt pile and started to dig a huge hole. Then I went to the tailgate and loaded up a little trailer with dirt. I could drive it all around the house. It was a cool tractor.

The Snowman

Matthew Clay
Wilson Elementary School, Grade 1

When I was four years old, it came a big snow. Me and my mom built our first snowman. He looked great. He had my mom's scarf on. I missed him when he melted. I am ready for another snow.

Jerdon's Incident

Andrew Cina
Lascassas Elementary School, Grade 6

On October 5, 2007 in Bridgeport, Alabama, a terrible and frightening incident happened to a seven-year-old boy named Jerdon Cina.

Jerdon and I were spending the day with our cousins riding four-wheelers on the farm. After a while, I was getting too hot and tired so I went in and watched TV to cool off. Jerdon got on one four-wheeler and our cousins got on the other. They headed off. They were riding to the top of the hill. My cousins quickly flew down the hill first, then Jerdon approached the hill. Our cousins were daring him to go down the hill.

At that moment he had a decision to make. He followed his cousins and flew down the hill, but at the middle of the hill he lost control and flipped. The four-wheeler fell on top of him. My cousins ran to help him. They put him on the back of their four-wheeler and took off towards the cabin.

When they got there, they took him off the four-wheeler and rushed inside.

After rushing in the house, my cousins and grandmother put him down on the bed. They tried to cool him off. Jerdon was lying on the bed saying that our cousins were praying all the way to the cabin. Moments later he was telling my grandma; that if, he was not a Christian he would have not been alive after the crash.

We picked him up and placed him in the car in order to head to Murfreesboro where we live.

When we arrived at our house my mother came rushing to the car, to help Jerdon to the house. Once inside my mom checked his stomach and decided to call the doctor, who immediately instructed her to get him to the hospital.

In the emergency room the doctors started to perform many tests. The results showed he had internal bleeding and a fracture in his lower back. He was then taken by ambulance to Vanderbilt Hospital for more testing. After a couple of hours, the doctor informed our parents that he would not need surgery but would be kept overnight for observation.

The following day the doctor told him he could go home, but he would not be allowed to engage in ANY physical activity for a period of thirty days.

Once they arrived at home Jerdon was tired but he stayed awake because the whole family was coming for the day to see Jerdon. We ordered pizza and celebrated that he was fine.

To this day Jerdon says he will never ride a four-wheeler or car again!

Nervous

Tyler Hendricks
Blackman Elementary School, Grade 2

I felt the butterflies flutter in my stomach as I stepped onto the stage. I began to giggle as I peered into the crowd. I recognized my mom sitting in the back row and the butterflies vanished from my stomach. I was not nervous anymore. When I got home, my mom and I snuggled on the couch because I did a great job.

Treasures

Brittany Bain
Stewarts Creek Middle School, Grade 6

Treasures aren't just silver and gold.
They are memories that can be new or old.
They could be memories of all the fun you've had,
Or even a couple of times that were bad.
So, whenever you're lonely or sad,
Don't be blue.
You'll always have your memories with you!

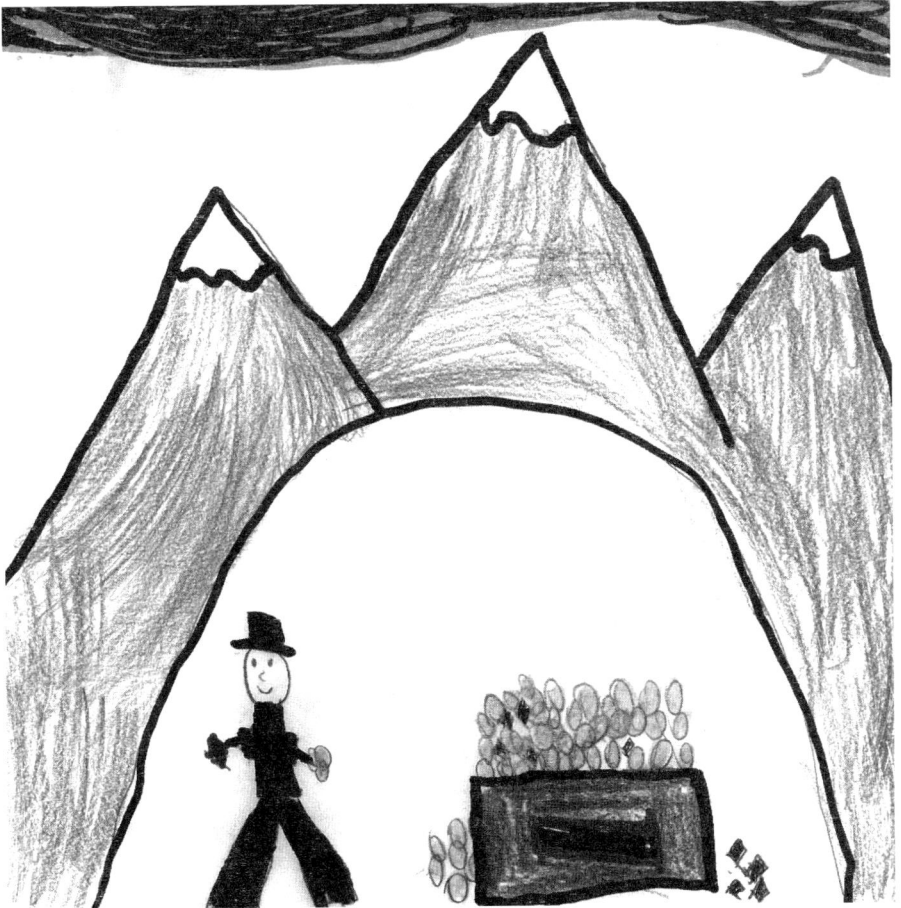

Teagan Paukner, Thurman Francis Arts Academy, Grade 2

Vacation

Cassi Clark
Smyrna High School, Grade 12

The sound of the waves,
The sand in my toes,
The feel of salt water
Getting up my nose.
Trying to body surf
And having no luck,
Riding in the back
Of a pickup truck.
Taking a walk
Just as the sun goes down,
Finding a sand dollar
Perfectly round.
Building a sand castle
With seashells on top,
Going out with family
To a souvenir shop.
A vacation like this
Is perfect in every way,
If only life could be like that
Every day.

The Night My Life Changed: When Katrina Hit New Orleans

Byron Pleasant
Oakland High School, Grade 11

On the night of August 29, 2005, my sister woke us up because she had found a little water on the floor. My step-dad said "It's ok, go back to sleep." A little later, more water came in our house and my step-dad said for us to get on top of the stove, refrigerator, dresser or anything we could get on. He also told us not to plug anything in because we might get shocked. The water kept coming in all night long. We could hear all kinds of sounds outside. Windows were breaking and water was rushing into our house. It was too deep to try and get out. My mom was on the stove and we were all scared we might die. I fell asleep on the counter and when I rolled over, I fell right into the water. I was dreaming I was in my bed asleep. I fell into the deep water in my house and almost drowned. I was cold and scared. My little sister started crying and my mom kept telling her it would be ok. The water started to go down and we thought it was over; but then the water came back even deeper. We tried several times to open the doors but the water pressure was to too much. We got hungry and we had no food. My daddy got some cans and he had to open them with his knife. He tried to get us to eat cold green beans or corn. It didn't taste good so I wouldn't eat it at first. But when I got hungry enough I did eat some of the cold food. I put hot sauce on it to help it taste better. The food in the refrigerator was bad.

We saw and heard people on their roofs yelling for help. We couldn't get to our roof. My step-dad knocked a hole in the wall trying to get some air in the room. It was hot and we were all tired of the water. We could hear helicopters outside and we tried to flash our flashlights to let someone know we were in the house and we needed help.

We saw an old man walking in the deep water and he just died. He died right in front of my house! I saw old people in the water that didn't make it. It was hard seeing the bodies. We saw trash floating in the water. The water was so nasty. We were trapped for three long days in my house in the water. A neighbor had a boat and he offered to take us to my school. He said you don't want to stay in your house. It is not going to get any better soon. Another neighbor wouldn't leave her home. She said she was going to stay with her house. I don't know if she made it out or not.

I don't know where my friends are. Are they ok? Did they get out? No one knows. The neighbor let us off and said we could walk the rest of the way to my school. Everyone was stealing clothes and food. It was wild! We heard people saying it was a free shopping day. We were hungry and wet. We needed food and clothing. I know stealing is bad, but we had nothing and we had to have food and clothing to live. I loved living in New Orleans. I had never been anyplace but New Orleans. This had been my home, but we knew we had to leave the house or die. The neighbor took us to my school. C. Colton Middle School in New Orleans' 9th ward. In New Orleans we have parishes not counties. In New Orleans we have areas called wards. I lived in the 9th ward. It was hit the hardest by the hurricane. In my school, we were dry and comfortable. Everyone was getting along.

It was like a big family. We had blankets, food, and sleeping bags. They found barbeque, soft drinks, and other food from the cafeteria. We got to sleep in the teacher's lounge. They had couches and chairs. It was nice to sleep on something soft and dry again. Everyone treated each other well. I felt safe and warm for the first time in days.

My family was safe and together. At least my Mom, step-dad, sisters, and I were safe. We did take food from the vending machine to eat but we didn't take the money. Everyone was stealing cars but my momma said no to that. We didn't know where anyone else was. I was barefoot and my step-dad got me some shoes. We heard about people in the Super Dome. We heard they were being stabbed and killed at the Super Dome. We heard that some were raped. We were glad we were safe at my school. The reports were also that people were dying on the streets. We had no power at the school. We talked to each other and that is how we passed the time. We always knew the levees could break but we never thought is could be this bad. We have flooded in the past but the water always goes down. I wondered if the water would ever go down. It seemed there was too much water everywhere. I wondered when we could go home. We were in the school for about three days. A Greyhound bus picked us up and took us to another bus that took us to the airport. We got in line to get on the plane. You couldn't take any alcohol so my step daddy had to throw his away because you couldn't take it on the plane. The plane was full with everyone trying to leave New Orleans. The plane landed in LaVergne, Tennessee. They had us stay in the barracks on the Army base. The women had to stay in one place and the men stayed in a separate place. They woke us up early to feed us and send the kids to school. They made us go to school. The school system got us clothes. I liked it at LaVergne High School. I met several people who were nice. I met a girl that liked me. We felt like we were settled. Then we were told we had to move. We moved to this apartment in Murfreesboro, Tennessee. They told us I would be going to Oakland High School. I had to start over again making friends. I still wonder where my friends are and if anyone has moved back. My teacher has tried to contact my old school trying to get information, but no one has answered her e-mails.

This is the second anniversary of when Katrina changed my life. Katrina is the hurricane that changed my life in New Orleans forever. I still want to go back some day and I will! And we all know New Orleans will come back better than ever.

Acknowledgements

Barfield Elementary School
Karen Myers
Sheralee Riddle

Blackman Elementary School
Tammy Anselmo
Libby Black
Kimberly Christopher
Wendy Davenport
Bonnie Eblen
Kelly Held
Kelly Henry
Catherine Herbert
Melnequa Holloway
Kelly Jones
Lynn Kennedy
Kim Marable
Pam Morgan
Krissa Seifert
Michele Slusher
Angie Smith
Wendy Spivey
Felicia Thompson
Connie Wiel
Rebecca Wiese
April Williams
Fannie Williams
Wanda Williams
Ashley Winrow
Kerri Womack
Evelyn Wray

Blackman High School
Peggy Nelson

Blackman Middle School
Paige Barber
Melissa Ball
Leisa Barrier
Leigh Anne Brown
Susan Lewis
Bridgette McCord
Paula Renfroe
Mary Ellen Zimmerman

Buchanan Elementary School
Suzan Warren

Cedar Grove Elementary School
Crystal Brown
Gena Capps
Kristen Conte
Kara Mullican
Angela Pope

Central Middle School
Beth Clark
Lisa Murphy

Christiana Elementary School
Erin Dwyer
Deborah Henderson
Christy Mann
Lora Vetter
Misty Waddell

Christiana Middle School
Melanie Bowen
Monica Everett
Lisa Ezell
Carol Haislip

Daniel McKee Alternative School
Pat Smith

David Youree Elementary School
Angela Montgomery
Melissa Smigielski

Eagleville School
Beverly Noland Barnes
Laura Bingham
Melissa Broyles
Theresa Hill
Carla McElwee
Nancy Warden

Holloway High School
Jennifer Williams

Homer Pittard Campus School
Nancy Perdue
Holly Ray

Kittrell Elementary School
Mary Merrill

Lascassas Elementary School
Amy Arriola
Becky Deaton
Tina Elms
Jennifer Frazier
Christina Harlan
Melissa Kincaid
Wanda Locker
Brenda Martin
Christina McAlexander
Shan McCormick
JoLyn McWhorter
KathyWest

LaVergne High School
Valerie Lay

LaVergne Lake Elementary
Beth Lewis

LaVergne Middle School
Billy Anderson
Tarron Huddleston

LaVergne Primary School
Cynthia Roberts

McFadden School of Excellence
Debra Brown
Christa Campbell
Christy Moore
Vanessa Tipton

Oakland High School
Lisa Beasley
Gina Blackburn
Tim Coffey
Jim Gifford
Eileen Haynes
Nancy Jackson
Timothy Nance

Riverdale High School
Ruth Taylor
Lil Welch
Dr. Patrick White
Renessa Yokley

Rock Springs Elementary School
Jill McHenry

Rock Springs Middle School
Deborah Hunt
April Sneed

Rockvale Elementary School
Linda Blanton
Stephanie Mattox Elliott
Shawn Lee
Ann Patient
Mary Patterson

Roy Waldron School
Dr. Margaret Guitard

Siegel High School
Kim Cing
Eileen Haynes
Belinda Juergens
Matt Marlatt
Trish Morgan
Kelli Nichols
Steve York
Barbara Zawislak

Siegel Middle School
Teri Beck
Sandra Boyd
Amanda Cheuvront
Nancy Sanders

Smyrna High School
Jennifer Ebert
Chrissy Grisham
Kris Pollack
Jill Walls

Smyrna Middle School
Stacey Bryan
Michelle Burke
Leslie Duke
Deborah Shipley

Smyrna Primary School
Tanya Chavez
Diane Giles
Kevin Gladish
Melanie Hatcher
Leonora Washington

Smyrna West Alternative School
Devin Dodson
Elizabeth Jennings

Stewarts Creek Elementary School
Jennifer Johnson
Heidi Redmon

Stewarts Creek Middle School
Anna Duncan
Jane Macomber
Beverly McGee

Stewartsboro Elementary School
Patsy Newberry

Thurman Francis Arts Academy
Shanya Caldwell
Nancy Essary
Rosanna Heard
Susan Loveless
Shannon Marlin
Beth Tuverson

Walter Hill Elementary School
Emily Baker
Teresa Brockwell
Karen Burrell
Beverly Carlton
Gina McClanahan
Dana Palmer
Mary Powers

Wilson Elementary School
Caren Davis
René Davis
Jacci Hooper
Joyce Hugle
Rhonda Lackey
Rachel Peay